AUTISM

CD

Protocol

... and other autoimmune disorders.

KERRI RIVERA

D.HOM

AUTISM CD
Protocol
...and other autoimmune disorders

KERRI RIVERA
D. HOM

Author: Kerri Rivera
www.kerririvera.com
kerri@kerririvera.com

Text editing:
Kerri Rivera

Cover design:
Maria Davila
Yonely Davila
@Davsamedia

Illustrations
Maria Davila
@Davsamedia

ISBN: 979-8-33037-862-3

First Edition
United States, January 2024

Copyright © 2024 Kerri Rivera

Published by Indy Pub

PARENT GUIDE

Empowering Parents on the Path to Autism Recovery.

*Step by step of the Kerri Rivera protocol by
Kerri Rivera for you.*

Kerri Rivera – D. Hom

DEDICATION

This book is the result of 20 years that I have been in the university of autism. The how to heal the damage that is autism. I feel that until we can recover 100% of the children 100% of the time, I will still be searching for additional answers. My mission in the autism recovery efforts began March 12th of 2004. That was 20 years ago. It is so hard to believe that it has been so long. Over these 2 decades I have had to opportunity to work directly and indirectly with over 100,000 families. The knowledge and experience that I have gained over these years has benefitted so many. The past 14 years of seeing the benefits of CD added to the biomedical protocol has been uplifting. Watching families apply my CD protocol and getting their children back makes me so happy and shows that I am on the right track. I am grateful to the families who have trusted me as well as those who have recovered their children and continued on to help others coming up behind them. Parents of recovered children inspire the other parents like nothing else can. I am forever grateful to the families who continue to stay in touch with me as their children who have since recovered go on to have other firsts in their lives like getting their driver's license and graduating high school as well as going on to university. This gives me the strength to continue forward and help the next generations of children whom will go on to do the same as these recovered individuals. This 2024 book of the CD protocol is for those who need it and want it. It is the book that many have desired to have. I will continue to research and update as changes for the better happen. I wish for every family that their dreams and prayers are answered. And that no other family ever has to suffer alone the sadness of the diagnosis of the autism spectrum disorder.

DISCLAIMER

The information presented in this book has been obtained from authentic and reliable sources. Although great care has been taken to ensure the accuracy of the information presented, the author and publisher cannot assume responsibility for the validity of all information or for the consequences of its use. Before initiating or applying any recommendation given in this work, we suggest that you first consult with a specialist or physician you trust.

INDEX

WHO IS
Kerri
Rivera?

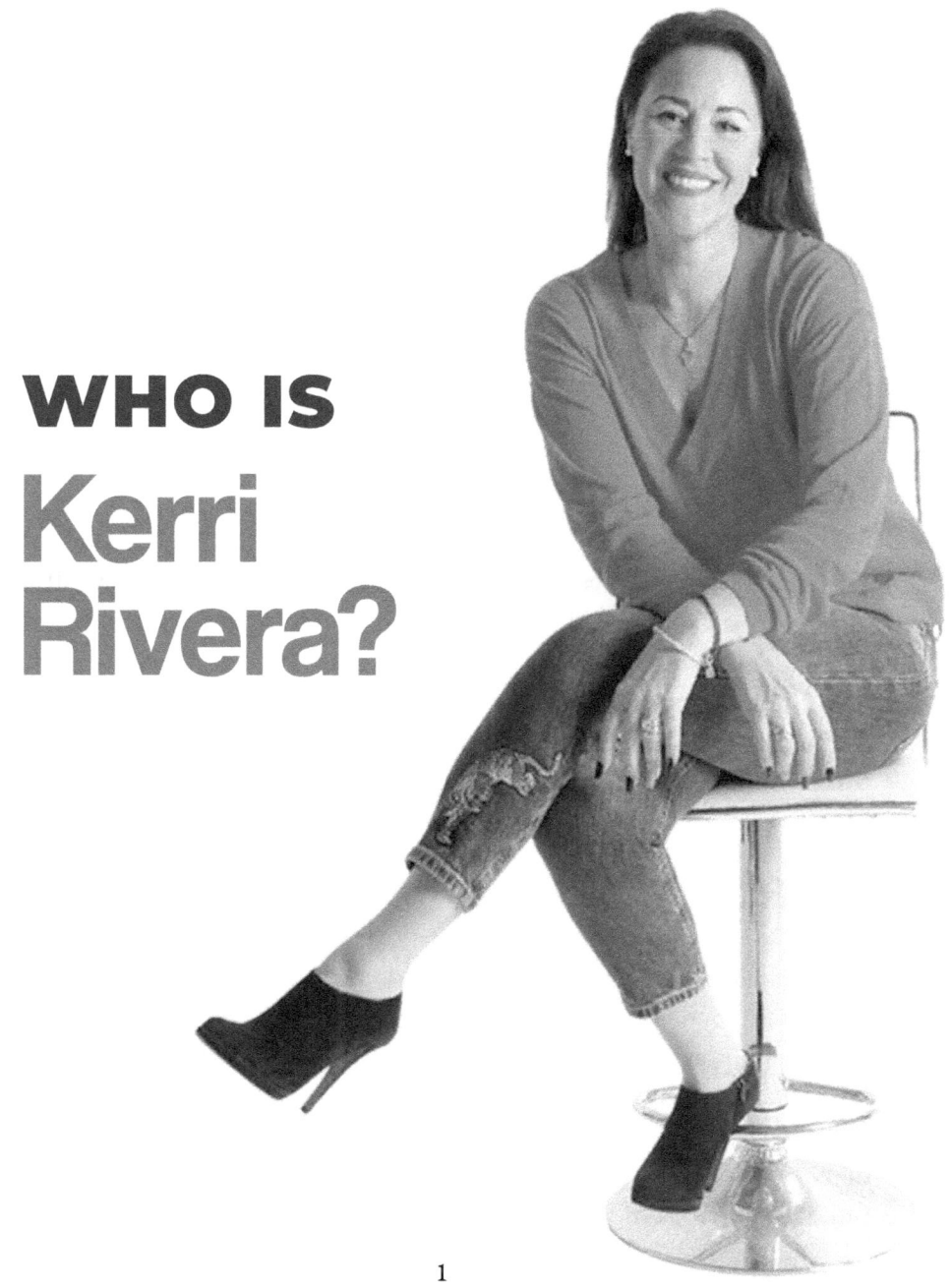

CHAPTER 1

Who is Kerri Rivera?

On March 12, 2004, my life changed forever, a day that will remain etched in my memory forever. It was the day when my son Patrick was diagnosed with autism, news that changed the direction of my life and sparked a tireless search for answers. Patrick came into the world healthy and full of vitality, like any other child. However, after a series of vaccinations during the first year of life, his health began to fade; he lost the skills he had developed such as speech, eye contact, interest in others, and more. The regression was devastating: his progress was fading, and my mother's heart was filled with anguish and sadness of a great loss, like mourning.

Despite seeking help from various doctors and trying many protocols. Nothing seemed to have a positive impact on Patrick's health, which continued to worsen as time progressed. When I realized that no one knew how to treat autism, even though I spent fortunes with so-called "professionals/doctors." It was in the midst of this darkness that my determination to find a solution on my own emerged. I realized that I can only count on myself to help my son. The "professionals" were only managing the symptoms of autism. But the full recovery that I was search for, they were not able to attain.

My first steps in helping Patrick focused on diet. A friend lent me a book about a diet for autism and Attention Deficit Hyperactivity Disorder (ADHD), which discussed the importance of a gluten- and casein-free diet. Without wasting any time, I decided to adopt this diet. Patrick's situation was challenging, as his food preferences had narrowed to dairy, wheat, and pure junk food. Wheat and dairy-based products were their favorites such as bread, flour tortillas, quesadillas, and pasta. Potato was the only gluten and casein free option he ate. For this reason, I began making homemade French fries that were fried in coconut oil and served with sea salt, as it was the only thing that aligned with his prior diet.

I removed everything that had gluten and casein from one day to the next. He ended up eating potatoes for several weeks without accepting to eat any other types of food and he was getting better and better every day. After only 3 days of implementing this dietary change, something extraordinary happened: Patrick spoke his first three words in more than a year. Patrick went from a 100+ word vocabulary at 1 year old to completely non-verbal at 2.5 years old. It was at that moment that I knew we were on the right track with improvements just by changing the diet to gluten and casein free he began to speak again.

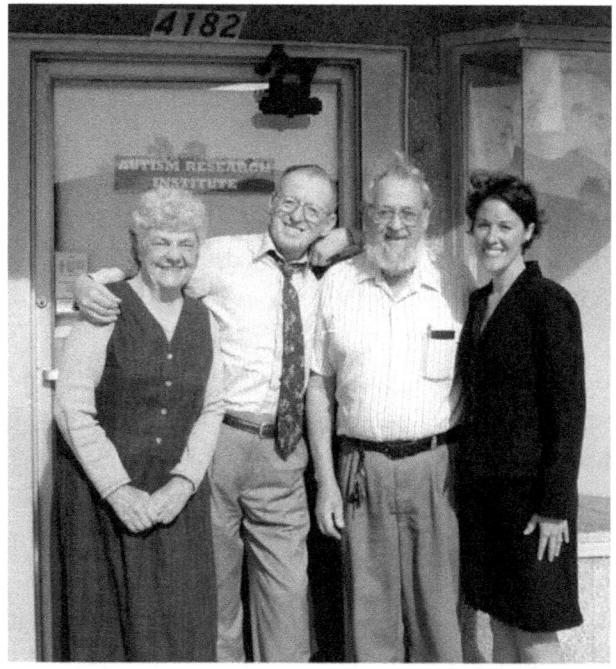

Mrs. Gloria Rimland, Bob Sands of Sands hyperba-rics, Dr. Bernard Rimland and Kerri Rivera

In 2006, I was blessed to meet Dr. Bernard Rimland, Ph.D., who is considered to be the pioneer of biomedical treatments for autism. In 1964, Dr. Rimland wrote the book CHILDHOOD AUTISM: THE SYNDROME AND ITS IMPLICATIONS FOR A NEURAL THEORY OF BEHAVIOR. This book changed the way the world viewed autism. Before his book, those in psychiatry thought that autism was caused by the "refrigerator" mother. In other words, it was the mother's fault who did not give love and attention to her child. Obviously, this was not true. But, before Dr. Rimland's book in 1964, they believed that this was the situation. Dr Rimland believed that something wasn't right inside the children which had nothing to do with the parenting skills of the mother. My meeting with Dr Rimland became the starting point of my mission. From Dr. Rimland, I learned invaluable lessons that marked the beginning of the direction in my approach. Dr. Rimland asked me over lunch in January 2006 to translate the DAN protocol! into Spanish and then to take the message of autism treatments to Latin America. He invited me to train as a DAN! doctor/clinician which I did for 4 years, from 2006 to 2009. I shared my desire to help other families. That's how Dr. Rimland entrusted me with the task of translating the DAN! protocol book (now called MAPS) into Spanish, a responsibility that I assumed with humility and determination.

Finally, in August 2010, I found a light at the end of the tunnel. Patrick was 10 years old, and I had been fighting for his progress since 2004. Words that had been elusive for him began to flow after a crucial discovery, Chlorine Dioxide (CD). On the first day of full dosing for his weight, Patrick began to say complete words of everyday things, such as "I want to go to sleep" at a suitable sleep time, "I want to take a bath," "I want to play blanket," "I want to brush my teeth," etc. From then on, his progress was more and more typical. I was able to enjoy his sincere smiles and hugs as well as many other things like him asking for kisses from mommy. The veil of autism was removed from his eyes. His improvements never faded. He has been back ever since. And my search for solutions has not stopped and each day the pieces of the autism puzzle fit together better. There is no age nor level of autism that cannot be improved.

Never think that there is a golden window of opportunity as some say. Until the day we die there will always be improvements if not the full healing (PC term for the c word).

Never think it is too late to help your child. Until the last day of his or her life there will always be an opportunity to get better or to make a full recovery.

I firmly believe that autism is treatable and that hope, and full healing prevails even in the darkest of times. During these two decades that I have been in the world of autism, my dedication has been focused on researching how we can support the body's natural healing processes. By addressing medical conditions that impact the gastrointestinal, immune, and metabolic systems in children with autism, autistic behaviors begin to fade and all of the systems in the body begin to work as they were supposed to again.

My path has been marked by the acquisition of knowledge and experience in various areas, including my Doctor of Homeopathy degree.

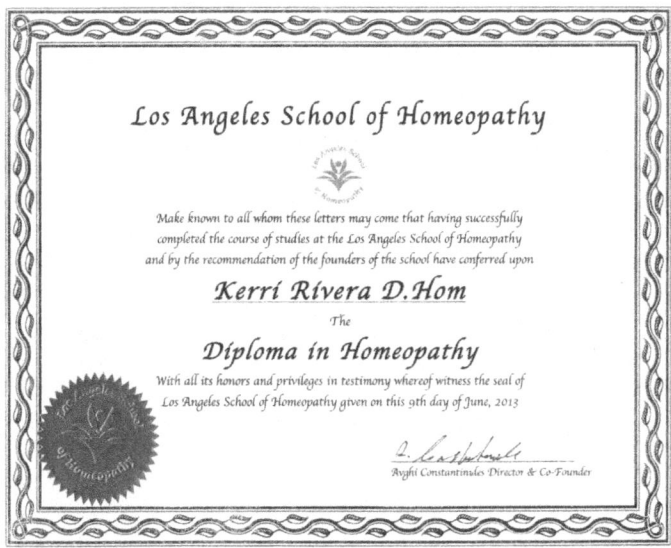

My certification as a DAN clinician! (now MAPS) by the Defeat Autism Now Foundation started by Dr. Rimland in 1970.

CME CREDIT CERTIFICATE

The Institute for Medical Studies
in Joint Sponsorship with

The Autism Research Institute

Verifies the attendance and successful completion
of the Autism Research Institute - Defeat Autism Now!
sponsored clinicians' seminar.

Level 1 Clinician Seminar
May 21-22, 2009

Kerri Rivera, medical director

has completed up to 13 hours of category 1 CME credit through
participation in the Autism One Conference
May 21-24, 2009 in Chicago, IL.

This CME activity has been planned and implemented in accordance with the
Essential Areas and Policies of the Accreditation Council for Continuing Medical
Education (ACCME) thru the Joint Sponsorship of the Institute for Medical
Studies (IMS) and the Autism Research Institute.

IMS is accredited by the ACCME to provide continuing medical education
for physicians.

IMS designates this educational activity for a maximum of 13 hours of
AMA PRA Category 1 Credits™. Physicians should only claim credit
commensurate with the extent of their participation in the activity.
Please retain this Certificate for your records.

The Institute for Medical Studies
14 Monarch Bay Plaza, Suite 202 Monarch Beach, CA92629

Certificate# 000566175

Autism Research Institute
4182 Adams Avenue
San Diego, California 92116

BERNARD RIMLAND, Ph.D., Director

419-281-7165
fax 619-563-6840
www.AutismResearchInstitute.com

November 2, 2006

To: Kerri Rivera

I would like to congratulate you on starting a DAN!-oriented clinic in Mexico.
Autistic children and their families will benefit enormously from your hard
work and dedication.

Thank you Kerri. Your efforts are welcome and appreciated.

Bernard Rimland, Ph.D.
Director

Technician in the management of hyperbaric chambers, director, and founder of the first biomedical clinic dedicated to autism treatments in Latin America in 2006, and my contribution as a pioneer in the use of CD to treat the symptoms known as autism. Nobody before me used the CD for ASD. Not even Jim Humble had experience with CD and ASD. Jim used to say that the trolls on social media hated me more than him because I work with children. Sadly, that was the case. But the families with the children who recovered their health love me. That is all that matters. Results matter, the rest is just background noise.

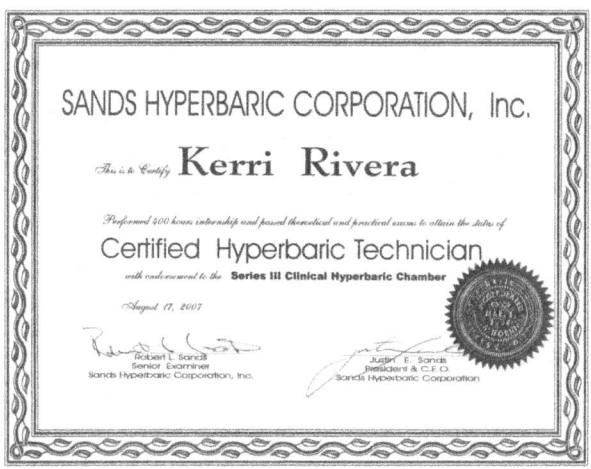

Through my books such as "Healing the Symptoms Known as Autism," "A Modified Ketogenic Diet," "First Aid," and "Low glutamate diet cookbook" I have shared my findings and experiences to guide others on their own journey. Since then, my role as a speaker at the largest international conference called AutismOne has allowed my message to transcend borders. I have presented at conferences in many countries on several continents such as the United States, Puerto Rico, Venezuela, Dominican Republic, Colombia, Bulgaria, Czech Republic, Spain, Turkey, and Mexico. Through these conferences, I have conveyed a message of hope, conveying my firm belief that there is hope and that autism is successfully treatable. **I know because I have seen it over and over again with my own eyes.**

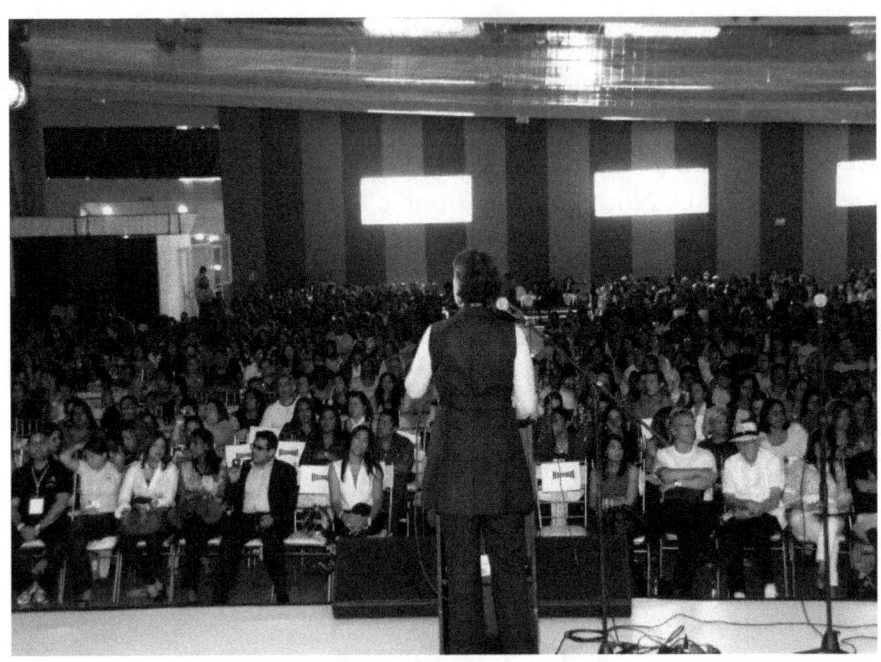

Kerri Rivera (from the back), Dr. Anju Usman, Andreas Kalcker, Jim Humble
III International Congress Overcoming Autism (October 2012, Venezuela)

In February of 2012, I started a movement on Facebook where we supported over 60,000 families in over 12 different languages in the various different groups doing my protocol. Unfortunately, Facebook has since put in place lot of censorship. So, the groups promoting the use of CD successfully for autism or anything else, would get canceled. They closed my page and all my groups related to my page overnight in February of 2019. I woke up without any groups when I had many groups in 13 languages with 60 moderators with more than 60,000 members between them. It was shocking and saddening to see the level of censorship that we are under as well as the lengths that they will go through for you not to learn about CD. Now however, we are on Telegram, Instagram, TikTok and soon I will be on more and more platforms with freedom of expression, perhaps a private platform, which I will give you information about very soon. If one day you can't find me on any of them. Send me an email to **kerri@kerririvera. com** and I will let you know where you can find me and the groups.

I do not feel that social media is stable regards to people speaking about health freedoms and certainly not those explaining how to use CD.

From this platform, I want to share the findings that I have acquired in my 20 years of experience. Knowledge is power and my mission is to empower people to make informed decisions and not waste time on misguided interventions that don't work. If you need help on this path, I want you to know that you are not alone. As a mother and specialist on the subject, I offer you my hand and I will not let you go until you reach your goal. Recovery is possible! Accept nothing less.

Kerri Rivera

Chapter 2
What is Autism?

- Autism according to Biomedicine
- PANDAS/PANS/PITAND
- My son was diagnosed with autism, where do I start?
- ATEC

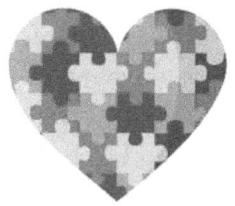

What is Autism?

A simple definition for autism is a developmental disorder that impairs the ability to communicate and interact among other problems.

The ATEC (Autism Treatment Evaluation Checklist) test is very good for understanding where children are on the spectrum. ATEC 0-10 is no autism. ATEC 30-160 is autism. ATEC 10-30 is ADD/ADHD or details to complete recovery. However, the goal is an ATEC of 0.

The term Autism Spectrum Disorder (ASD) usually includes the following diagnostic terms:

• Pervasive Developmental Disorder (PDD)
• Pervasive Developmental Disorder Not Otherwise Specified (PDD-NOS)
• Autism
• Atypical autism
• Asperger's syndrome
  PANDAS/PANS/PITAND
• High Functioning Autism (HFA)

Autism according to biomedicine

Autism is a spectrum disorder, meaning it appears in a variety of forms and levels of severity. Some people develop typical abilities in terms of speech and language, or develop exceptional abilities, but struggle with social and behavioral differences. Others may have communication problems, sensory sensitivities, and behavioral problems, such as obsessive compulsive disorders (OCD), tantrums, repetitive behaviors, aggression, and self-harm. The good news is that appropriate treatments get rid of these. The more we get rid of these. The faster we get to the ATEC of 0.

Almost 100% of children diagnosed with autism today are born healthy and without autism. Then something happens to their immune system in the first 24 months of age that they start to get sick, then become disengaged, lose speech they had, or show severe problems with behavior and focus. And shortly after they are diagnosed with "autism." Yet no one understands what has happened to their child? Parents lose their children who were previously completely healthy, loving, interactive, verbal, and connected to their environment. In most cases it takes place over a period of time. They don't typically fall into autism overnight. In some cases, after a surgery, the child can come out of the anesthesia having lost eye contact, speech and/or social behavior. They can begin to show signs of autism right after having anestesia.

Autism today is an epidemic of diseases of the immune system, caused by toxins in our environment, excess pathogens, excess heavy metals, food allergies, leaky gut, inability to detoxify, oxidative stress, inflammation among other things. The result is a toxic load in our children's bodies that prevents their immune system from working properly. This situation worsens with the presence of viral infections, heavy metals, parasites, bacteria, and fungi that stress the immune system, creating allergies, gastrointestinal problems and serious inflammation in the brain, affecting the areas of communication, language and social interaction.

The medical community in general still has the idea that autism is a psychiatric disorder and indicates for us to medicate our children with psychostimulant drugs. What they really need is treatment to deal with illnesses caused by autoimmune disorders. It has been discovered that by treating the serious, underlying medical conditions in the gastrointestinal tract, immune and metabolic systems that children with autism have. The autistic behaviors begin to disappear. The children begin to regain their lost skills, as their bodies heal. It is time to look at our children's behaviors as a way of expressing the physical ailments or underlying conditions that they have. Autism does not respond to psychiatric drug treatments. The pharmacological medications do not improve the conditions of the symptoms of autism. They can only put a bandaid over them, yet they correct nothing. Stop the meds, the symptoms return. Since the underlying cause never went away.

Every child with autism is different. However, some behavioral patterns have been established that can guide us. If your child has some, most or all, of the following behaviors, you should take the ATEC and start this protocol as soon as possible:

1. Loss of verbal or physical skills.
2. Echolalia: constantly repeating the same thing or repeating what one hears (phrases or words). Like when they answer you with the same question you asked or repeating the words you just said.
3. Seems as if they were deaf. However, they do not tolerate certain loud sounds such as that of a blender or the microwave.
4. Does not make direct eye contact.
5. Obsessing with certain objects for no reason.
6. Does not show interest in toys or does not use them properly.
7. Carries a toy or an object from one place to another without meaning and/or without using them properly.
8. Tends to gather objects by lining them up or stacking them up to form a tower.
9. Shows disinterest in their environment, family and/or in social interactions with others.
10. Doesn't respond to their name.

11. Does not obey or follow instructions.
12. When they want something, they do not ask for it nor point to it. Yet they take someone else's hand directing them to what they want. Many times, they push the person's hand to the cabinet or wherever the object of desire is.
13. Reject physical contact. Don't like to be touched, hugged, or picked up. Preferring to be left alone.
14. Flapping hands like a flutter (as if trying to fly) rhythmically and frequently.
15. Spins, rocks, or swings on their own.
16. Twirling or flapping objects.
17. Standing still and looking at a point as if hypnotized.
18. Walking on tiptoes (as if doing ballet).
19. Can be hyperactive (very restless) or hypoactive (extremely lethargic).
20. Shows aggression towards others or maybe self-injurious (hitting oneself) at times. They can push, pinch, or squeeze as well.
21. Is obsessed with order and routine, rejects change.
22. Gets very angry and has tantrums for no apparent reason or because they didn't do something that they typically do.
23. Has episodes of laughter for no apparent reason. Can go from maniacal laughter to crying with tears for no apparent reason.
24. Extremely advanced in some skills, such as patterns, shapes, or numbers, while others may be non-existent.
25. Does not seem to acknowledge the presence or feelings of others.
26. Does not seek comfort in times of sorrow or pain.
27. Does not imitate nor perform imaginary activities, such as pretending to be a character or person.
28. Wants to eat only certain foods in particular and reject others. Can be textures of the food or the types of food. Some will only eat blended or pureed food. Some prefer dry and crunchy. Some sweet or savory.
29. Does not tolerate certain textures as in clothing as well as in foods. Can cause fear or nausea just by seeing these foods or articles of clothing. Just to see or feel a texture in food can cause the child to vomit as a nausea reaction.

(30) Suddenly, run without fear of danger nor without stopping. It is known as fight or flight.

Based on new discoveries, a series of physiological symptoms that were not previously considered are now added to this list of behaviors. These symptoms have been found highly associated with autism and are key to observing a complete clinical picture of the child and thus receiving effective treatment. It is common for children diagnosed on the autism spectrum to have:

(1) Constipation, diarrhea, or both.
(2) Food allergies, especially dairy and wheat as well as with other high glutamate foods.
(3) Some types of dermatitis, eczema, or other skin issues.
(4) Doesn't sleep well or may have trouble falling asleep.
(5) May have reflux, hiccups, or gastritis. Some hold food in their mouth after chewing for a long time. Some may even vomit food that has been chewed and swallowed back into the mouth later.
(6) Distended tummy.
(7) Dark circles under the eyes.
(8) Seems to feel no pain when something hits him or when the child falls down.
(9) They may have a cough or croup.
(10) Might have an immediate negative reaction to vaccines.
(11) Viral infections.
(12) Stop talking after being vaccinated or have a seizure after a vaccine.
(13) Constantly have nasal allergies, sinusitis or respiratory infections.
(14) Recurring ear infections.
(15) Suffers from asthma.
(16) Severe mouth ulcers.
(17) Low muscle tone.
(18) Difficulty holding a pencil or crayons.
(19) Big head.
(20) Problems walking well as if dizzy.
(21) Issues with fine motor and/or gross motor skills.

15

An official diagnosis is not necessary. The ATEC and symptoms are enough to know that action must be taken.

PANDAS/PANS/ PITANDS

PANDAS: It is an acronym for Pediatric Autoimmune Neuropsychiatric Disorder Associated with Streptococcal infections. PANDAS/PANS/PITAND are autoimmune disorders triggered by a streptococcal infection, in which antibodies attack the brain and cause neuropsychiatric conditions. Bacterial hijacking of the cells will occur. The antibodies trigger an immune reaction that damages these tissues, causing joint pain due to the antibodies. When the basal ganglia of the brain are affected, they are believed to be responsible for OCD movements that occur in TICs. The TICs are sounds or movements that cannot be controlled and happen with frequency.

PANS: Pediatric Acute onset Neuropsychiatric Syndrome
PANDAS/PANS/PITAND all have similarities to Tourette's syndrome. The symptoms may come and go and appear suddenly. There is a high rate of Obsessive Compulsive Disorder (OCD) and/or Tourette's syndrome among relatives of children with PANDAS/PANS/PITAND.

PITANDS: PITAND are infectious triggers of PANS, including viruses, Lyme, chicken pox, and mycoplasma.

IS PANDAS/PANS/PITAND THE SAME
AS STREP THROAT?

No, strep throat is an acute, short-term illness. Throat swab testing for "strep throat" (streptococcus) is NOT a test for PANDAS/PANS/PITAND. PANDAS/PANS/PITAND are chronic disorders that consist of streptococcal bacteria in the intestine and in the blood. Testing for strep, even in blood tests, is unreliable. In most cases the tests come back negative. Even if the person has symptoms of PANDAS/PANS/PITAND.

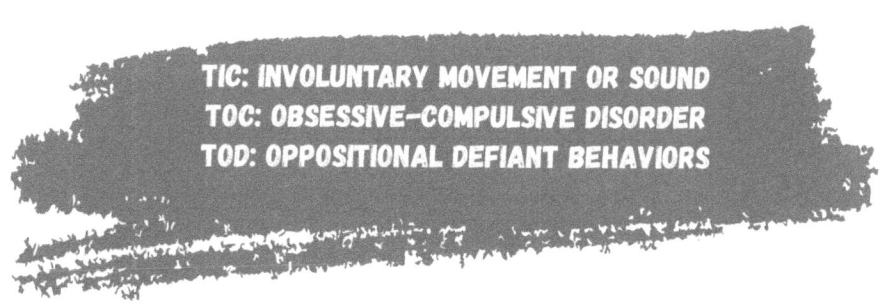

TIC: INVOLUNTARY MOVEMENT OR SOUND
TOC: OBSESSIVE-COMPULSIVE DISORDER
TOD: OPPOSITIONAL DEFIANT BEHAVIORS

The 5 official diagnostic criteria for PANDAS/PANS/PITAND are:

1. The presence of TICs and/or OCD.
2. Typically, the neuropsychiatric symptoms begin before or around puberty.
3. Sudden onset of symptoms with episodes of exacerbation interspersed with periods of partial or complete remission.
4. May have an association between symptom onset or exacerbation of symptoms due to prior streptococcal infection or another acute illness in their environment.
5. Adventitious movements such as motor hyperactivity, choreiform movements during symptom exacerbation.

There may be an association between the onset or exacerbation of symptoms due to a previous streptococcal infection or other acute illness in your setting.

Adventitious movements such as motor hyperactivity, choreiform movements during exacerbation of symptoms.

WHAT ARE STREPTOCOCCAL BACTERIA (STREPTOCOCCUS)?

Streptococcus bacteria are an ancient organism that survives in the human host by hiding from the immune system. They hide by arranging molecules on the cell wall so that they appear almost identical to the molecules found on heart tissue, joint tissue, skin tissue and brain tissue. This concealment is called "molecular mimicry." This allows the streptococcus bacteria to evade detection by the immune system for a long time. However, the molecules of the streptococcal bacteria end up being recognized as foreign by the body and the person's immune system reacts to the molecules by producing antibodies. Due to the molecular mimicry of the bacteria, the immune system reacts not only to the strep molecules, but also to the molecules of the human host that were mimicked. Antibodies attack molecules that mimic the person's own tissue. These antibodies that react to both molecules of the strep bacteria and similar molecules found in other parts of the body are an example of "cross-reactive" antibodies.

Studies from the National Institute of Mental Health and other agencies have shown that some cross-reactive antibodies target the brain causing OCD, TICs, and other neuropsychiatric symptoms of PANDAS/PANS/PITAND.

Laboratory tests of blood and throat swab are not helpful as they rarely find what is there when it comes to strep. Throat swabs are not intended to test for systemic and chronic PANDAS/PANS/PITAND. The best test is the observation of symptoms. I would always believe the child and their behaviors over a negative lab test.

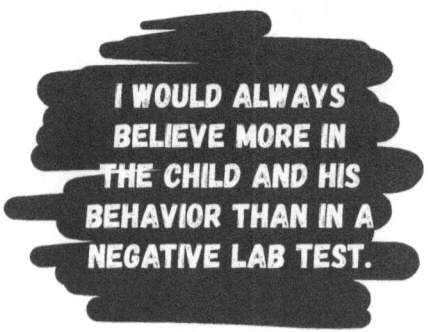

I WOULD ALWAYS BELIEVE MORE IN THE CHILD AND HIS BEHAVIOR THAN IN A NEGATIVE LAB TEST.

WHAT ARE THE SYMPTOMS OF PANDAS/PANS/PITANDS?

To have **PANDAS/PANS/ PITANDS** you can have some and not all of the symptoms:

The symptoms are:

> TIC: INVOLUNTARY MOVEMENT OR SOUND
> OCD: OBSESSIVE COMPULSIVE DISORDER
> ODD: OPPOSITIONAL DEFIANT DISORDER

» • OCD/Obsessive Compulsive Disorder
» OCD with different types of food, restrictive to smell, taste, texture that may cause vomiting or wrenching upon the sight of the food or nausea when the texture of food is in the mouth etc.
» OCD repetitive movements and/or behaviors.
» OCD routines as in sameness and patterns.
» Fear.
» Anxiety.
» Separation anxiety.
» Depression.
» Bedwetting/enuresis even into the teen years and/or frequent urination.
» Panic attacks.
» TICs which are involuntary movements or sounds.
» Emotional lability.
» Irritability.
» Oppositional Defiant Disorder (ODD).
» Academic decline with onset of symptoms.
» Sensory or motor difficulties.
» Sleep disturbances.
» Tourette's syndrome or Tourette's like behaviors.
» Memory problems.
» Inability to concentrate.
» Joint pain.

- » Almost catatonic state.
- » Incessant screams.
- » Night terrors.
- » Fine motor impairment, such as a change in handwriting
- » Apparent sensitivity to light, sound, and touch.
- » Fury.
- » Hyperactivity.
- » Emotional and/or developmental regression.
- » Visual or auditory hallucinations.
- » Sensory issues from having contact with tags from clothing or seams in socks.
- » Better at home than in school or other places where there are more variables and changes.
- » Might have a particular attraction to one parent or caregiver. Being very upset if they leave.
- » Better with adults than with other children. Adults are far more predictable than children are. The people with PANDAS/PANS/PITAND will be more comfortable around predictable environments as well as predictable people.

WHAT ARE THE TRADITIONAL TREATMENTS MODALITIES FOR PANDAS/PANS/PITAND FROM THE MEDICAL ESTABLISHMENT?

- » Behavioral therapies.
- » SSRIs (psychotropic medications).
- » Antibiotics.
- » IVIG (intravenous immunoglobulin).
- » NSAIDs (nonsteroidal anti-inflammatory drugs).
- » Tonsillectomy.
- » Corticosteroids.

None of these will heal, recover, nor cure. PANDAS/PANS/PITAND. Most only suppress and further damage the body. So many of the children on the ASD do poorly with pharmaceutical medications.

That is partly what will lead to a further regression into the disease after one of these medical treatments.

WHAT HAS WORKED AND WHAT CONTINUES TO WORK FOR PANDAS/PANS/PITAND?

- » CD
- » Black Seed Oil
- » Berberine
- » Diet (low glutamate)
- » Mebendazole
- » Structured Silver

Can you recover from PANDAS/PANS/PITAND with this protocol?

Yes, of course!

My son was diagnosed with autism. Where do I start?

It is essential that you understand that you are not alone in this. My team and I are here to provide you with the help and information you need on this journey. Remember that knowledge is the most powerful tool to help your child regain their health. Get informed and start the path to recovery. Autism is preventable, treatable, and recoverable!

In this book, I will provide you with the essential steps to follow for my CD Protocol. Thanks to my experience having worked with over one hundred thousand families around the world, thousands of children have recovered. Yes, recovered! They no longer have autism, nor do they have autistic behaviors that limit their potential. Tens of thousands if not more have had a notable improvement in their quality of life as well.

When one recovers from autism, they are the same as the other typical children who have never had autism. You cannot tell who had autism and who didn't.

Before starting the protocol or any protocol for that matter, I recommend that you complete the ATEC (Autism Treatment Evaluation Checklist) form at _www.autism.org._ The ATEC is in about 20 different languages. The ATEC is one of the most widely used assessment tools in the autism community. This screening test was designed by Dr Bernard Rimland and is for parents to track their child's progress over time and evaluate the effectiveness of treatments.

By completing the ATEC, you will gain a solid understanding of your child's current symptoms, which you can discuss with me and/or your child's therapists. This form will provide you with a reference point using measurable numbers as to where your child is on the autism spectrum. This will allow you to assess which areas of development he or she is making progress in and where he or she may need more support. This also helps to know what supplements to add or other treatments to begin.

The score obtained on the ATEC will reflect your child's level of need. The higher the score, the more severely impacted by autism. If the ATEC score is less than 10, it will indicate that there are no symptoms of autism, just a little room for improvement. The goal is to reach an ATEC 0. An ATEC of zero/0 means that there are no issues whatsoever. There is no autism, no ADD nor ADHD. There are no longer social issues, speech issues, behavioral issues nor physical issues.

To follow your child's evolution, I suggest you take the ATEC at the beginning of the protocol and then repeat it every 3 months till we reach an ATEC of 0. The ATEC is free and easy to use. You can find it at: www.autism.org

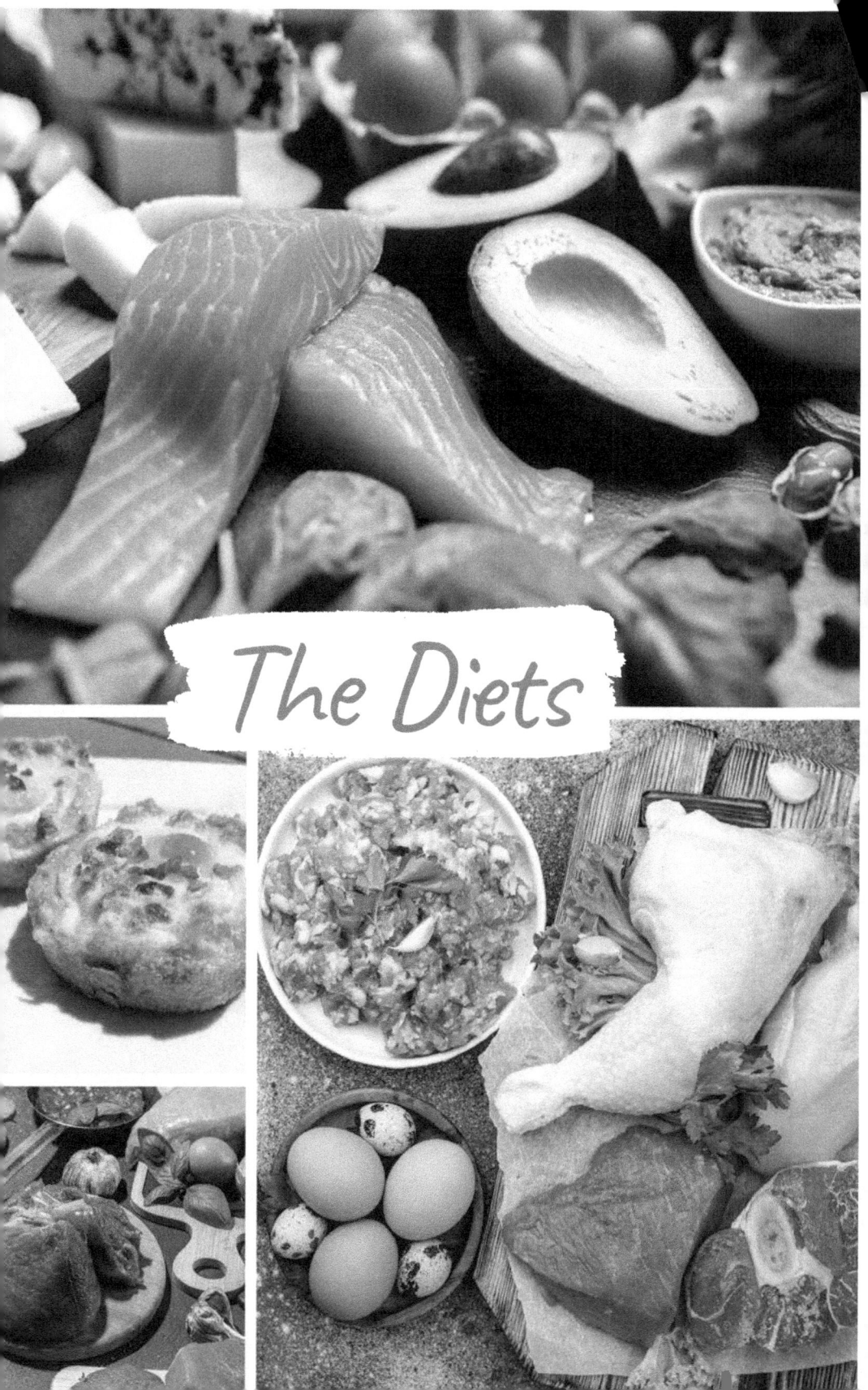

The Diets

Chapter 3
The Diets

- Carnivore Diet
- Modified Ketogenic Diet
- Low Glutamate Diet

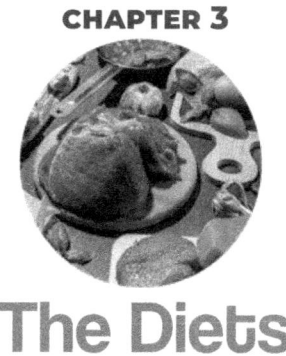

The Diets

Carnivore diet

The carnivore diet is the ancient way of eating. This means it simulates the diet that our ancestors evolved from by eating a carnivore diet for over 3 million years.

About 10,000 years ago, at the dawn of agriculture, human beings had not eaten a diet based on plant foods, grains, nor cereals. These elements were not part of the human diet until only about 10,000 years ago. The grain and cereal diet are a diet based on dollars and cents. It is cheap and easy to feed many people on grains and cereals. It is not a healthy diet. But it is good for keeping hungry, poor people alive. Now they have tried to make it fashionable to eat these nutrient poor foods since they do not have our best interest in mind. The meat and good fats were kept for the ruling, wealthy class. Not for us so called useless eaters. Whatever they say is good or bad the opposite is usually true.

The main objective of the carnivore diet is to obtain all the necessary nutrients through foods of animal origin. Generally, it involves eating a variety of meats, such as beef, lamb, goat, chicken, pork, fatty fish, casein-free clarified butter (Ghee), tallow (beef fat), lard (pork fat), duck fat and eggs.

"Animal fats are nutritious, muscle protein, and meat-specific micronutrients are the foundation for our healthy cellular structures and energy, hormonal regulation, cognitive vitality, and mental health. Animal fats help to reduce inflammation in the human body.

Plant based foods, on the other hand, expose our bodies to a long list of stressors such as excess fiber, excess carbohydrates, natural anti-nutrients as well as plant toxins, toxic molds and industrial pesticides, all of which harm body tissues and promote chronic inflammation, the root of modern diseases."

By Dr. Kiltz

WHAT FOODS ARE ALLOWED
ON A CARNIVORE DIET?

When you start the carnivore diet, you'll be surprised at how simple, yet satisfying your shopping list becomes. So much less planning and cooking that those other less healthy diets.

Marbled meat (fatty): Most carnivore diets focus on ruminant meats (beef, lamb, goat, deer, elk, etc.) including fatty cuts such as ribeye, New York strip, brisket, ribs, skirt steak, flank steak, 50/50 ground beef to fat, lamb, pork belly as in bacon without chemicals. No cold cuts nor packaged meats like bacon and ham.

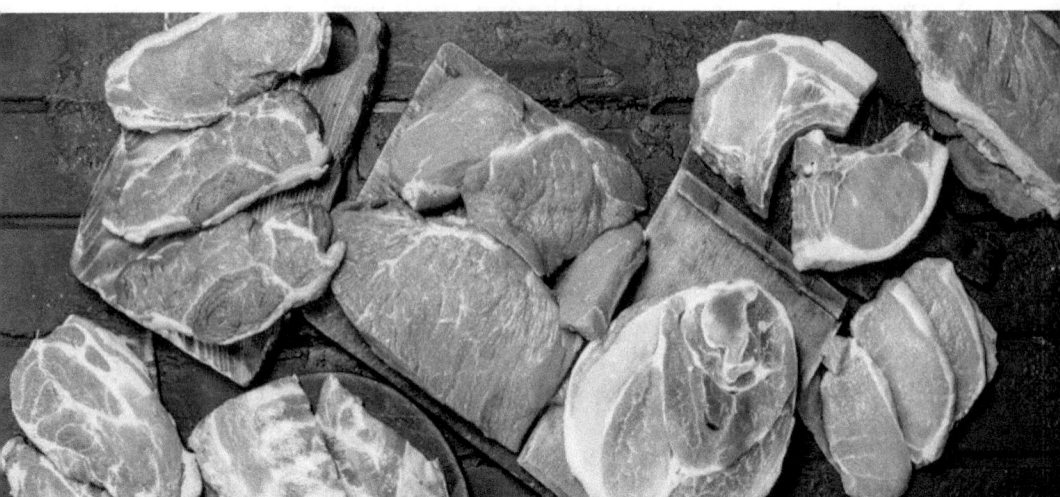

Animal fats: Since a carnivore diet is a high fat, zero carb and a moderate protein diet. All your meats should have 1 to 2 tablespoons of casein free ghee, beef tallow or lard if there is not much fat in your protein.

Eggs: Eggs are packed with a near perfect blend of fats, proteins, and vitamins. Hard boiled eggs are a fantastic carnivorous snack when you're on the run.

Fatty fish like Atlantic mackerel, anchovies, king salmon and arctic char provide omega-3 fatty acids, as does ghee. Ghee is clarified butter. Make sure that you use one that is certified casein free ghee.

Seafood: Opt for wild salmon, shrimp, and squid instead of farmed raised ones, as the latter are usually fed soy and corn. It is important to note that some farmed seafood may contain antibiotics and other medications added to the water to prevent illness in fish and shellfish in the farm tanks. An additional suggestion is to cook them with casein-free ghee to increase the fat percentage.

Add enough salt to all your foods to provide your body with important electrolytes. Sea salt or pink Himalayan salt are a good option. Make sure that your salt does not have any fluoride added. We all need to take Humic/Fulvic no matter what.

Important note: It is important to note that a carnivore diet is inherently a ketogenic (zero carb, moderate protein, and high fat) diet. On a carnivore diet, the body will make energy from fats. Fat is a much cleaner fuel for the brain and body that sugars/carbs. It is such an easy diet to follow. Simply focus on fatty meats and cook with plenty of animal fats. It is so easy.

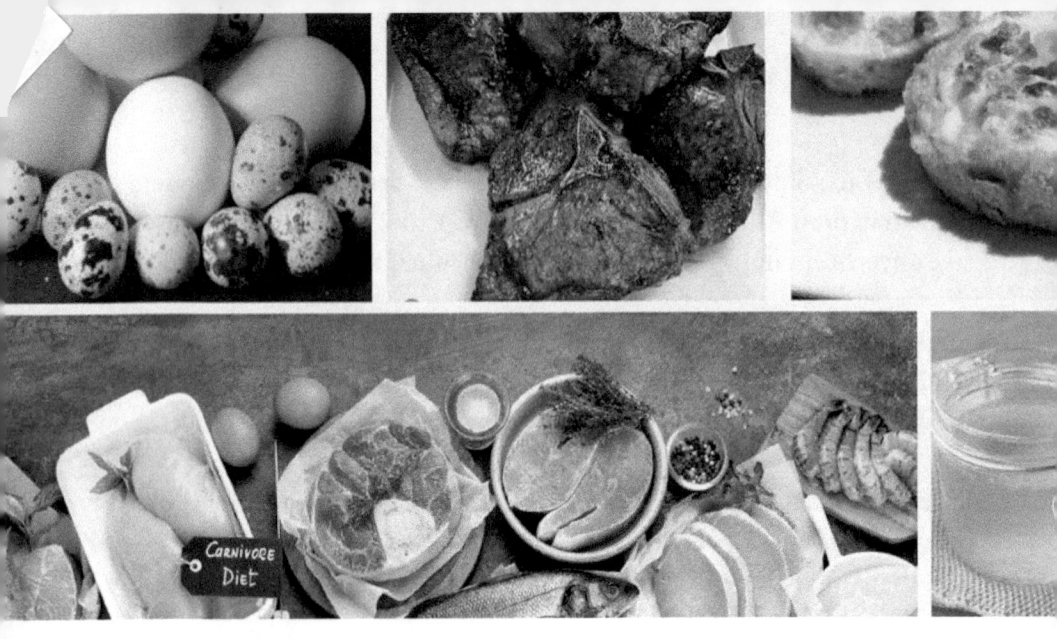

HOW CAN I START A CARNIVORE DIET?

Depending on previous dietary history, some people may start the diet right away, while others will benefit from a transition strategy. People who have subsisted on a high carb diet and a processed food diet will need to segue into the carnivore diet sttarting slowly over a period of a few weeks. It is not that the carnivore diet is bad. It is that your body will be going through a type of detox and have withdrawal symptoms. We can actually become adapted to eating junk food and carbs. The body is such an amazing machine. It can survive on garbage as well as healthy foods. Obviously, illness will come to though who subsist on garbage as opposed to those who consume healthy foods.

6-WEEK TRANSITION PLAN:

Week 1:
3 low carb, 100% carnivore meals
8 low carb meals (Proteína animal + Vegetales)
Reduce fiber by 25%

Week 2:
2 days 100% carnivore meals
5 days of low carb meals (Animal protein + Vegetables)
Reduce fiber by 50%

Week 3:
3 days of 100% carnivore meals
4 days of low carb meals (Animal protein + Vegetables)
Reduce fiber by 75%

Week 4:
5 days of 100% carnivore meals
2 days of low carb meals (Animal protein + Vegetables)
Reduce fiber by 100%

Week 5:
6 days of 100% carnivorous meals
1 day of low carb meals (Animal protein + avocado, cucumber and/or lettuces)
Reduce fiber by 100%

Week 6:
You made it! You have made the transition to 100% carnivore. Congratulations!

From week 6 and beyond, human beings can eat 100% carnivore for their entire lifetime as we did for millions of years before the vegan/vegetarian fashion came into existence. In many cases the high carb, low to no protein diet was necessary to keep people alive.

Carbs may have their place in the food chain. Yet, if you are trying to heal the gut/brain connection. You will not have the same success as you would with a high fat, moderate protein and low to no carb diet.

WHAT SHOULD I DO DURING
THE ADAPTATION PERIOD?

Make sure you eat according to your body's desire and get enough rest. You can also add more salt, electrolytes, magnesium glycinate, and potassium gluconate. Make sure to keep the minerals and electrolytes balanced by taking humic/fulvic minerals. Avoid heavy exercise because it takes some time for the body to adjust to burning fat as fuel instead of glucose/sugar/carbs. As you adapt you will have more energy to exercise even more than before going carnivore. The transition can vary from person to person. While some have a very easy time and others struggle. The prior diet has a lot to do with the transition. If you had a pretty decent diet as in lower carbs and not a lot of processed foods in your diet. You can change from one day to the next without issue.

Detox reactions to a prior poor diet are called Herxheimer reactions. They may include fatigue, headache, malaise, low energy, insomnia, increased thirst or urination, changes in bowel frequency, constipation, diarrhea, joint or muscle pain, and rashes. Kerri Rivera and her team of moderators can help make the transition to carnivore easier. Basically, those who have had a high carbohydrate way of eating or consumed a lot of processed foods are the ones who might have Herxheimer reactions if not taking time to transition. Many have eaten high carb and/or processed foods for a long time. For them, it is not uncommon to have Herxheimer reactions to detoxing from toxic foods.

Herxheimer reactions resolve naturally within a few days or weeks. You will then start to see improvements in every aspect of your health including your energy, sleep, digestion, reduction of inflammation and more.

HOW LONG UNTIL I START SEEING RESULTS?

A few days to a few weeks. After the adjustment period, you will begin to see improvements in energy, sleep, mood, digestion, skin, speech, behavior, gut motility and more. We can see it reflected in the ATEC with the children. We did a small study with 40 families switching from the modified ketogenic diet for autism to the carnivore diet for 4 months. We had a 10% recovery from autism in this short period of time. The carnivore diet is worth trying. It can make the end of autism and the beginning of full healing like no other diet I have seen in 20 years in autism biomedical interventions. The results are so fast. The more carbs and processed foods in the diet. The longer the healing will take.

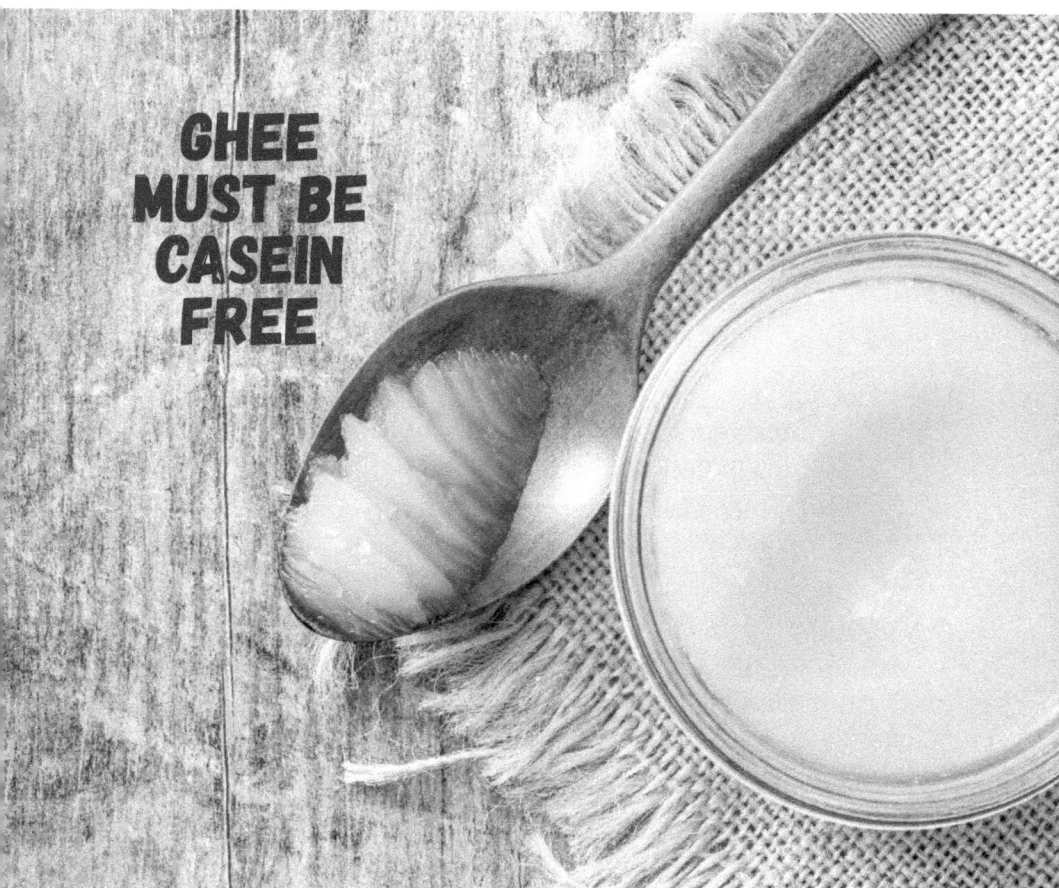

GHEE
MUST BE
CASEIN
FREE

Day 1:

» Breakfast: Scrambled eggs scrambled in the bacon fat with bacon.
» Lunch: Pork chops with ghee
» Dinner: Grilled beef filet and a cup of broth from the brisket

Day 2:

» Breakfast: Carnivore crepes and organic bacon.
» Lunch: Baked chicken thighs
» Dinner: Grilled pork ribs.

Day 3:

» Breakfast: Crispy organic bacon with hard boiled eggs.
» Lunch: Grilled salmon filet with ghee and a couple of crispy chaffles with ghee.
» Dinner: Grilled lamb chops with ghee and drippings from the lamb chops

Day 4:

» Breakfast: Poached eggs, strips of bacon on chaffles.
» Lunch: Beef burger and ground pork with ghee.
» Dinner: Grilled beef steak and a cup of brisket broth with some ghee melted in it

Day 5:

» Breakfast: Carnivore bread or cloud bread with scrambled eggs (scrambled in ghee or bacon fat) and organic bacon wi thout preservatives nor smoking.
» Lunch: Baked chicken with melted ghee on top and a cup of brisket broth.
» Dinner: Lamb chops with ghee and drippings

Day 6:

» Breakfast: Crepes made from egg with ground beef and organic bacon
» Lunch: Grilled salmon filet spread with ghee and a chaffle or 2.
» Dinner: Hard boiled eggs and brisket broth

Day 7:

» Breakfast: Chaffles with shrimp coated with pork rind flour fried in ghee.
» Lunch: Pork belly accompanied by hard boiled or poached eggs.
» Dinner: Brisket from the slow cooker/crock pot/express pot cooked for 4 to 5 hours

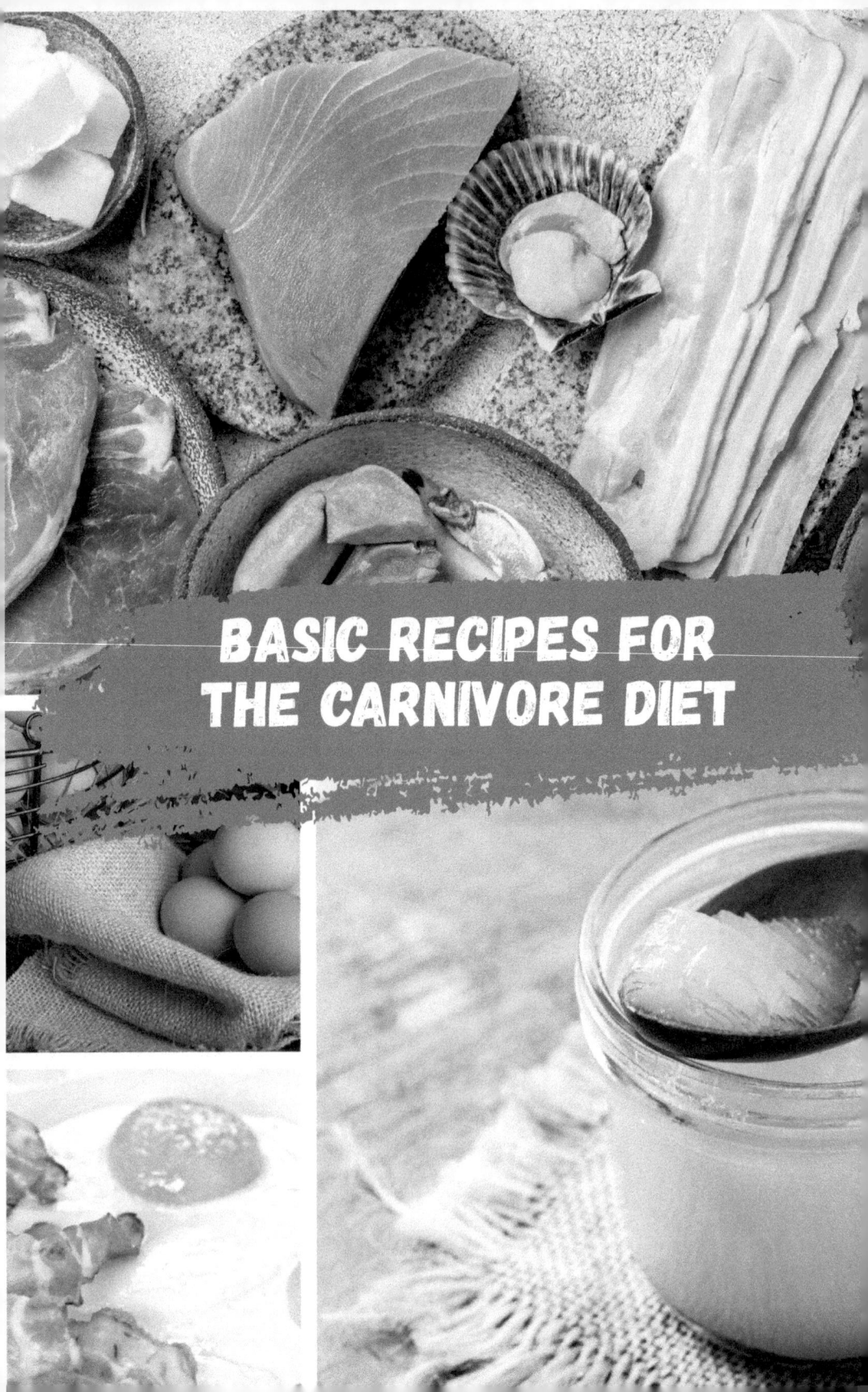

BASIC RECIPES FOR THE CARNIVORE DIET

BRISKET BROTH

Ingredients:

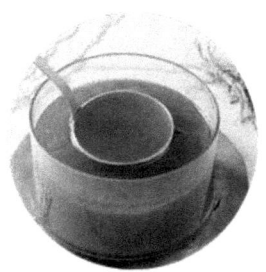

- » 1 brisket
- » 1 tablespoon of ghee
- » Himalayan pink salt or sea salt and pepper
- » Water

Instructions:

Spread ghee on the brisket with salt and pepper. Place it in a slow cooker such as a crock pot. Cover and simmer on high for between 4 to 5 hours. If you prefer, you can opt for a pressure cooker, where cooking is limited to a maximum of 30 to 40 minutes, and enjoy a broth full of good fat and quality protein. And you have the most tender and delicious meat.

CARNIVORE BREAD

Ingredients:

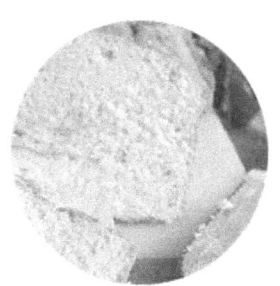

- » 250 grams of chicken or ground beef.
- » 4 eggs.
- » 2 tablespoons casein free ghee
- » Salt and pepper to taste.

Instructions:

Separate the whites from the yolks and beat the whites until there are stiff peaks. Mix the chicken or ground beef with the yolks, ghee, and add salt. Then, fold in the egg whites with gentle, folding movements. Place the mixture in a loaf pan and put it in the oven for 30 minutes on 300 degrees farenheit/148 degrees celsius.

CHAFFLES

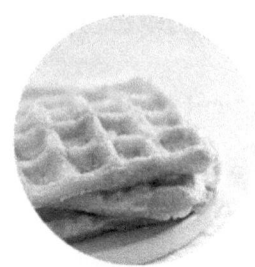

Ingredients:
- » 4 eggs
- » 2 tablespoons of Ghee
- » 2 pork rinds (ground)

Instructions:

Begin the process by grinding the pork rinds until they reach a flour-like texture in the blender. Then, add the eggs and ghee, and continue processing until you achieve a homogeneous and uniform mixture. Then, take portions of the dough and place them on a preheated waffle maker or griddle, letting them cook until they acquire an attractive golden hue and a crispy texture.

For the best results with this recipe, be sure to select bagged pork rinds. Before purchasing them, carefully check the ingredient list on the packaging. Ideal pork rinds should contain only pork skin and salt. Avoid those that have additional ingredients.

CLOUD BREAD

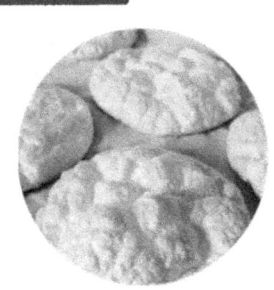

Ingredients:
- » 3 eggs
- » 1/4 teaspoon cream of tartar
- » A pinch of salt.

Instructions:

Preheat the oven to 150°C (300°F) and line a tray with parchment paper. If you have formed pans like a muffin pan or bun form pan it is better. Separate the yolks from the egg whites if you are not using the egg whites in the carton. In a separate bowl, beat the egg whites until peaks form.

Then, gently combine the beaten whites with ¼ tsp of cream of tartar and 1 whole egg, it will take less than 5 seconds with the hand beater to incorporate the cream of tartar and the whole egg to the egg whites. Shape into balls on the prepared tray with an ice cream scooper or use the form pans and bake for 30 minutes until the cloud bread is golden brown and firm to the touch. If you want a sandwich bread shape, place the mixture in a rectangular bread mold. Once baked, remove the cloud breads from the oven and let them cool completely.

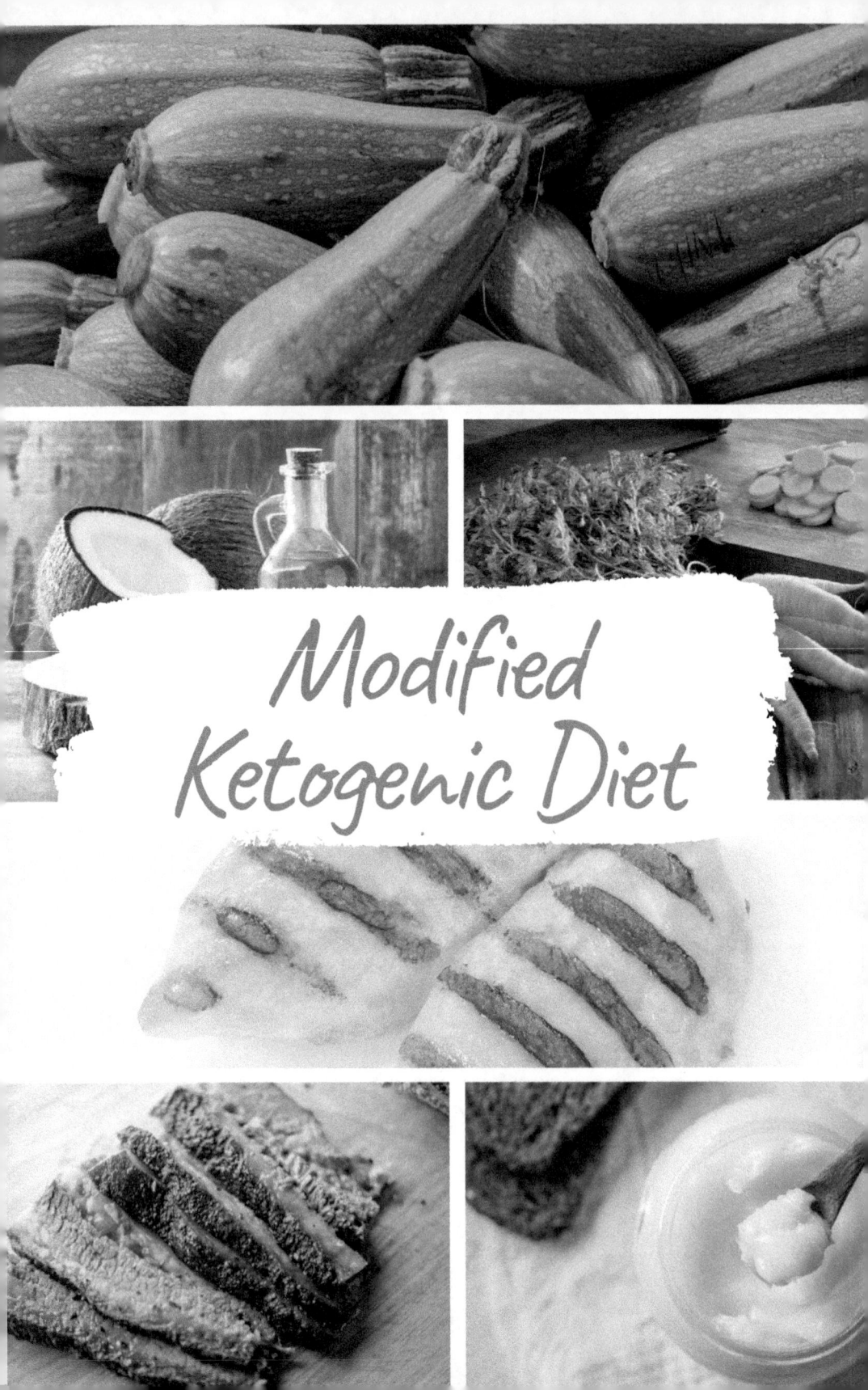

Modified Ketogenic Diet

Modified Ketogenic Diet

The modified ketogenic diet is based on a high fat consumption where 50% of calories are provided by good fats such as C8/MCT, coconut oil, olive oil, beef tallow, lard, and casein-free ghee. There are 2 grams of animal protein per pound of body weight and the rest in vegetables, some nuts and seeds as well as stevia or monk fruit to sweeten so that the body must resort to lipids as its first source of energy.

When you reduce carbohydrates and increase good fats, it causes your liver to increase the metabolism of body and dietary fat into energy compounds called ketones" or "ketone bodies." It is an alternative fuel for the body that is used when there is a shortage of carbohydrates (glucose) in the blood. Ketones help the body produce more energy by increasing the activity and oxygenation of mitochondria, providing better performance of brain cells and related mental functions.

ALLOWED FOODS

Animal protein: Beef, chicken (No chicken skin), turkey, lamb, pork, organic bacon (no preservatives), wild fish, seafood (limit your consumption and never eat farm raised, they must be wild), wild game meat, organ meats, eggs etc.

Fats and Oils: Coconut oil, MCT oil(C8), avocado oil, olive oil, casein-free ghee, lard, duck fat, and beef tallow

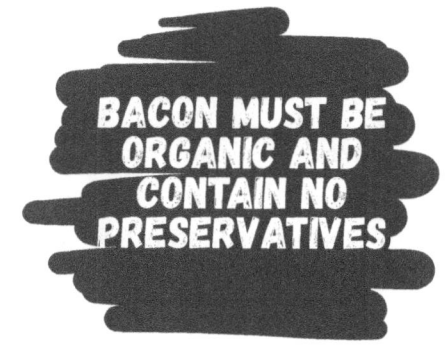

BACON MUST BE ORGANIC AND CONTAIN NO PRESERVATIVES

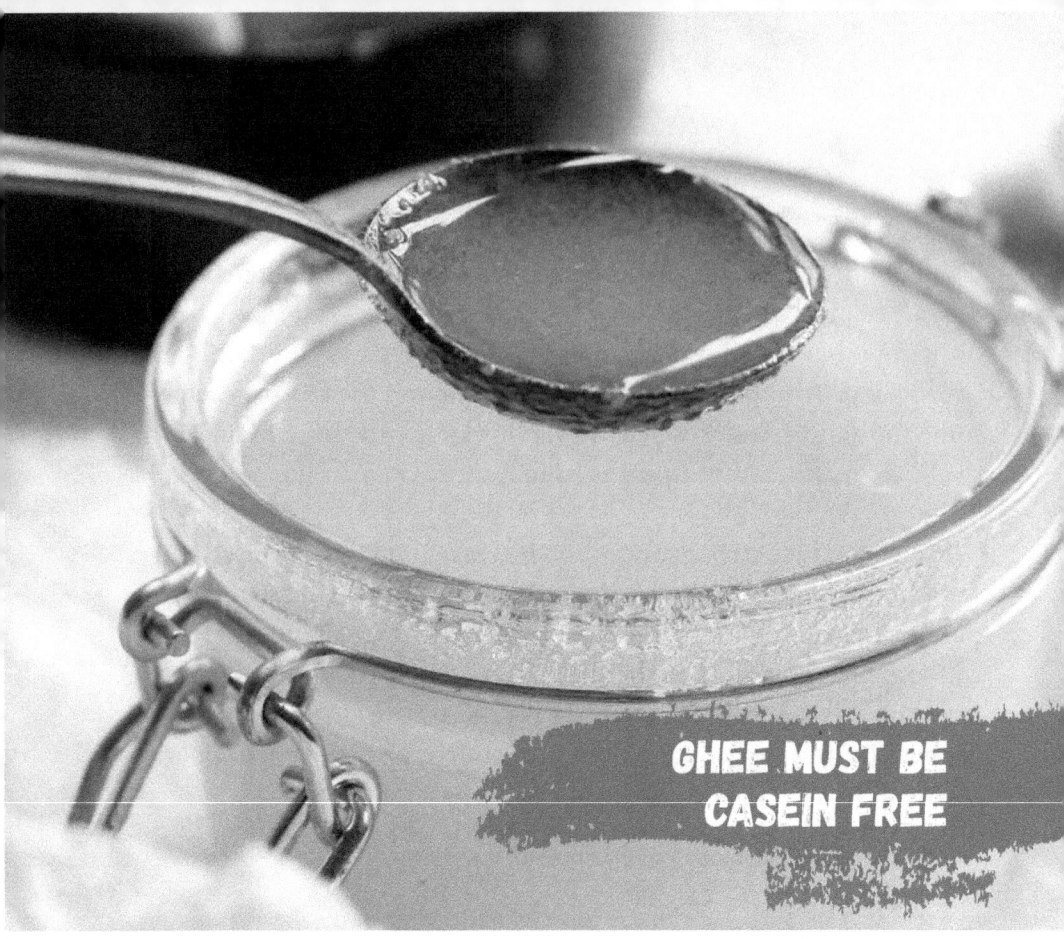

Vegetables: Asparagus, cabbage, cucumber, celery, kale, zucchini, lettuce, avocado (technically it is a fruit), turnips, parsnips, carrots, bell peppers.

Nuts and Seeds: Cashews, chestnut, hazelnuts, pistachios, coconut, macadamias, pecans, chia seeds, hemp seeds, sesame seeds either black or white, black cumin seed, flax seeds (linseed), sunflower seeds, pumpkin seeds.

Sweeteners: Stevia and Monk fruit

Others: Xanthan Gum, Baking powder (Aluminum free), Cream of tartar, Cinnamon, Vanilla (alcohol free), Pink Himalayan salt or sea salt.

C8/MCT
Medium Chain Triglycerides

In the modified ketogenic diet, fat consumption is essential. The ketogenic diet is characterized by being high in fat, moderate in protein and low in carbohydrates. Low carbohydrates would be under 50 carbohydrates a day at least. The main goal of this diet is to induce a metabolic state called ketosis, in which the body uses fat as its main source of energy instead of carbohydrates.

C8/MCT IS A SUGGESTED SUPPLEMENT WHEN FOLLOWING A MODIFIED KETOGENIC DIET

Ketosis is the metabolic state in which the body primarily uses ketones and fats as an energy source instead of carbohydrates. C8/MCT is especially necessary to help promote ketosis quickly creating ketones and helps raise blood ketone levels. C8/MCT has no taste or smell like other MCTs. You should always look for the MCT/C8.

A very common mistake parents make when implementing a low-carb diet is not including C8/MCT or increasing fat intake, which is very dangerous. Without carbohydrates and fats, the body will not have enough energy, which will lead to weight loss, weakness, and bad mood in the child. If your child does not tolerate or like fat, this diet may not be suitable for him/her at this time.

WITHOUT CARBOHYDRATES AND FATS, THE BODY WON'T HAVE ENOUGH ENERGY, LEADING TO WEIGHT LOSS, WEAKNESS, AND IRRITABILITY IN THE CHILD.

Age	Dose per day (ml)
2	60
3-5	90
6-8	105
9-10	105
11	120
12-13	120
14	135
15	150
16-45 and up	165

Suggestions:

The dose of MCT/C8 oil should be divided between the main meals (breakfast, lunch, and dinner)

Example: A person between 16- and 25-years old needs up to 165 ml of MCT/C8 or other fats per day. That means that you should distribute those 165ml between the main meals like 55ml with breakfast, 55ml at lunch and 55ml at dinner.

Although MCT/C8 is tasteless and odorless, its slimy texture may be uncomfortable for some people and may cause nausea. Therefore, it is not advisable to consume MCT directly in the mouth, as if it were a syrup. Instead, it is recommended to start with 1 ml diluted in coconut milk, soup, or broth. Then each day try to increase the dose of MCT/C8 a little more until reaching the dose according to age or tolerance.

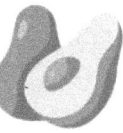

AVOCADO IS HIGH IN HISTAMINES AND MAY NOT BE WELL TOLERA-
TED BY SOME PEOPLE. SIGNS SUCH AS RED CHEEKS, RED CIRCLES
UNDER THE EYES AND EARS, IRRITABILITY, HYPERACTIVITY COULD
BE SYMPTOMS OF HISTAMINES. IN THIS CASE, CONSIDER ELIMINATING
AVOCADO.

Day 1:

  » Breakfast: Scrambled eggs with avocado and organic bacon
    free of preservatives and sugar.
  » Lunch: Chicken salad with lettuce, avocado, and cilantro
    olive oil dressing.
  » Dinner: Salmon filet with ghee and asparagus.

Day 2:

  » Breakfast: Scrambled eggs with chaffles
  » Lunch: Salmon salad with homemade mayonnaise, green
    beans, and cucumber.
  » Dinner: Chicken or turkey thighs with cabbage salad and
    grated carrots.

Day 3:

  » Breakfast: Scrambled eggs with sardines in olive oil.
  » Lunch: Chicken or shredded meat with allowedvegetables.
  » Dinner: Grilled beef filet with asparagus wrapped in
    organic bacon.

Day 4:

  » Breakfast: Eggs with ground beef mixed in it
  » Lunch: Lamb chops with lettuce, cucumber, and avocado
    salad.
  » Dinner: Grilled pork leg with Brussels sprouts sautéed in
    olive oil.

Day 5:

» Breakfast: Omelet with vegetables sautéed in ghee and some strips of organic bacon.
» Lunch: Chicken breaded with ground pork rinds served with cucumber and avocado.
» Dinner: Grilled salmon filet drowned in ghee with asparagus

Day 6:

» Breakfast: Egg omelet with bacon and avocado.
» Lunch: Ground beef meatballs with egg and avocado.
» Dinner: Grilled lamb chops with grilled asparagus and garlic butter

Day 7:

» Breakfast: Brisket from the slow cooker/crock pot.
» Lunch: Shrimp salad with lettuce, avocado, cucumber, and olive oil.
» Dinner: Beef filet with green beans sauteed in ghee.

Note: Keep in mind that you can adjust the portions based on your child's needs and preferences. Maintaining a proper balance between fats, proteins and vegetables is essential to following the Keto-Mato diet, a funny name that some parents have given to this diet and that makes me smile. Keto from ketogenic and Mato from glutamate. However, they are not wrong, as this modified version of the ketogenic diet is based on low glutamate vegetables, along with allowed fats, proteins, nuts and seeds. You have to remember that you have to count calories and carbohydrates. To be on a ketogenic diet, you should consume no more than 25 carbohydrates a day. I hope you enjoy it! Remember to include the portion of MCT/C8 according to your child's age or tolerance in each meal. There are a lot of things to take into consideration. It is important to do the best we can for them everyday. The better the diet, the faster the healing, the sooner the ATEC will reach 0.

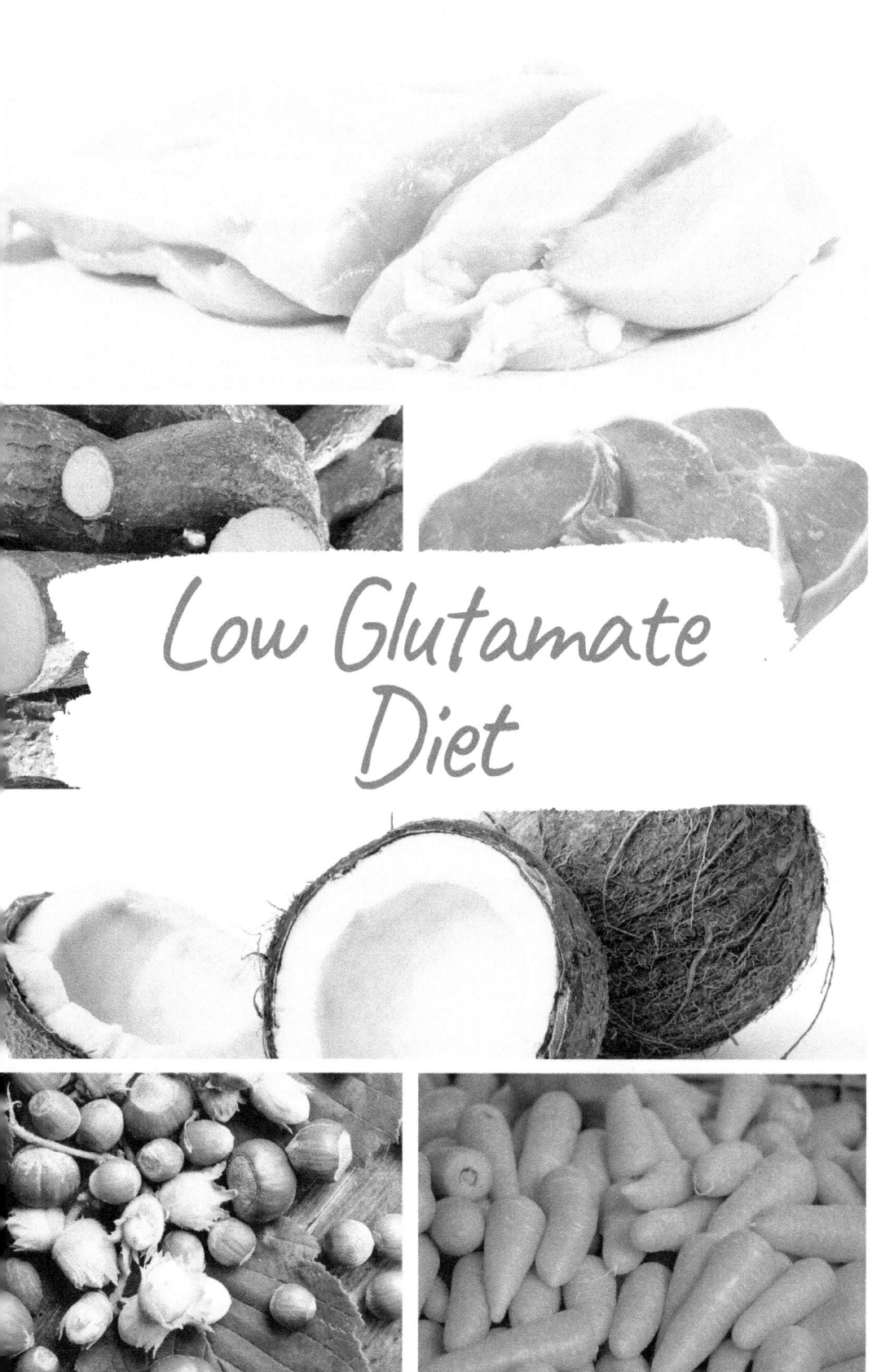

Low Glutamate
Diet

Low Glutamate Diet

The low glutamate diet was written and started by me in 2020. In 2020 I went back to the 1997 book by Dr Russell Blaylock named EXITO-TOXINS THE TASTE THAT KILLS. My shock was that this extremely important information has been around for 27 years. Glutamate is so damaging to the brain. Yet you don't hear "professionals/medical doctors" talking about it. If you go to a consultation with a biomedical autism doctor. You will be asked if you are doing a diet. If so, which diet. But they will never ever tell you how bad eating foods high in glutamate are for the brain. That said, here in my book you will be told things that you would not have heard before. Since no one is really interested in the full story. Autism is not from parasites. It is not always from vaccines. I have spent 20 years looking at autism, what it is, what it isn't and the solutions for full recovery. "The diet" is a HUGE piece of the recovery puzzle. Why is the carnivore diet successful in recovery of autism? It is a no glutamate diet. Families that cannot do the carnivore diet have to do the low glutamate diet. Otherwise, the brain will continue to be under attack by glutamate and the recovery will slip through your hands. You can do all the detox protocols that you want. But, if you are not aware of the glutamate in foods that occur naturally, you are basically shooting yourself in the foot before running a marathon. We need to get the diet piece right. I am very grateful for the work of Dr Russell Blaylock, and I am glad to be able to bring it to light so every year we get more and more children to the ATEC 0. This is my greatest wish. Full health and healing for all.

Glutamate and GABA are two chemicals in the brain that play opposite roles. Glutamate is excitatory and stimulates nerve cells, while GABA is inhibitory and calms them. A proper balance between them is crucial for the normal functioning of the brain and nervous system.

When there is excess glutamate compared to GABA, hyperstimulation of neurons can occur, resulting in cell damage and death. This situation can lead to neuronal dysfunctions, inflammation and oxidative stress, aspects associated with neurological and neurodegenerative disorders.

When someone has a leaky gut, which is the case for everyone on the autism spectrum. Those who have an ATEC above 10 have leaky gut problems. If you consume foods high in glutamate, you will have damage to the neurons because the glutamate leaves the intestine and via the bloodstream it reaches the brain where it causes problems as in neuronal death.

People with excess pathogens can develop hypersensitivity to glutamate, meaning that even low levels of this substance can trigger inflammatory responses. Foods with high glutamate contents, such as gluten, dairy, soy, corn, tomatoes, broccoli, berries, bananas, processed foods, etc. are damaging to the brain of people with leaky gut and autoimmune disorders. A low-glutamate diet can help normalize inflammatory signaling and keep glutamate levels low. Treating pathogens, eliminating heavy metals, and adopting a low-glutamate diet are essential to maintaining a healthy balance between glutamate and GABA. High glutamate foods will cause the blood brain barrier to become more porous allowing more glutamate, toxins, and heavy metals to get into the brain. Thus, causing more damage to the brain.

If we do not have a leaky gut, then the natural glutamate present in foods is not a problem. Higher than normal glutamate levels will cause a leaky blood brain barrier and neurons to start firing abnormally. At these concentrations the cells use the apoptosis process. The body cannot eliminate the amount of glutamate we consume. Glutamate crosses the blood-brain barrier. The blood-brain barrier will not be able to keep glutamate out.

Even as we age, the blood-brain barrier becomes more porous. There have been experiments that have shown that glutamate can open the blood-brain barrier on its own. Most symptoms are subtle and develop over time, such as ASD, dementia, Alzheimer's, and epilepsy. Food manufacturers have gone to great lengths to make sure dangerous glutamate appears benign; hydrolyzed vegetable protein, vegetable protein, caseinate, yeast extract, nutritional yeast, and natural flavors, to name a few.

Glutamate can be a flavor enhancer, in addition to being found in natural whole foods. They are not good for anyone.

The main culprit of course is synthetic MSG, which is found in processed, canned and cold cut foods. However, glutamate also exists naturally in certain foods. In a healthy individual with a healthy intestine, consuming foods containing natural glutamate does not usually cause any problems. However, in people with a leaky gut, natural glutamate can cause a lot of damage.

Glutamate is an excitotoxin which is a substance that literally stimulates neurons to death. This causes brain damage of varying degrees. This will affect physical and neurological health. Excitotoxicity is a process where nerve cells are damaged by excess stimulation of neurotransmitters such as glutamate. Excitotoxicity can cause encephalopathy and seizures, as well as other neurological symptoms such as ADD, ADHD, autism, PANDAS, PANS, PITAND, mood disorders, learning disabilities, Alzheimer's, strokes, and headaches. Processed foods have a huge amount of glutamate/excitotoxins. However, even in foods that were previously considered healthy, glutamate is present. We see this in broccoli, tomatoes, bananas, berries, and bone broth, just to name a few. Interestingly, foods containing glutamate are so addictive that the brain will literally crave foods that harm it. How can we protect our brains and the brain of those we love? Avoid all processed and packaged foods. Therefore, eat a diet of whole foods low in glutamate. Then once the leaky gut is sealed, the child will be able to eat whole foods with a high content of natural glutamate such as tomatoes and berries to name a few.

Animal protein:
Beef, chicken (without skin, chicken skin is high in glutamate), turkey, lamb, rabbit, duck, pork, wild salmon, shrimp, eggs.

Nuts:
Hazelnuts, cashews, macadamias, pistachios, coconut, pine nuts and pecans.

Seeds:
Sesame seeds of all colors, sunflower seeds, flaxseeds, chia seeds and pumpkin seeds.

Fats/oils:
Olive oil, coconut oil, lard, avocado oil, beef tallow, casein-free ghee, c8/mct.

Grains/legumes:
All lentils/beans/kidney beans are allowed, except not chickpeas/garbanzo, which are high in glutamate. Although grains and legumes are generally low in glutamate, it is recommended to limit their consumption due to their high carbohydrate content.

Fruits:
Cantaloupe, watermelon, pears, apples, peaches, nectarines, and apricots. (fruits are of limited consumption due to their high fructose content, which is sugar after all).

Tubers:
Potatoe, cassava, yucca.

Vegetables:
Carrots, asparagus, lettuce, celery, peppers, cucumber, zucchini, chayote, jicama, turnips, radishes, cabbage, brussels sprouts, nopales, green beans, avocado (technically a fruit).

AVOCADO IS HIGH IN HISTAMINES AND MAY NOT BE WELL TOLERATED BY SOME PEOPLE. IF YOUR CHILD EXPERIENCES PHYSICAL CHANGES SUCH AS REDNESS IN THE CHEEKS, RED CIRCLES UNDER THE EYES, RED EARS, OR BEHAVIORAL CHANGES SUCH AS IRRITABILITY OR HYPERACTIVITY, THEY MAY BE EXPERIENCING HISTAMINE-RELATED SYMPTOMS. IN SUCH CASES, CONSIDER ELIMINATING AVOCADO FROM YOUR DIET.

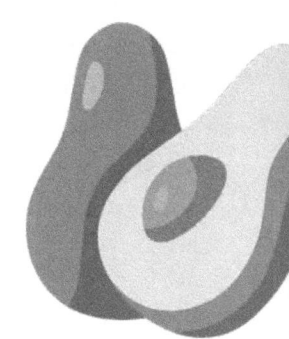

Cereals:
Rice, quinoa, arrowroot (limited consumption due to excess carbohydrates).

Sweeteners:
Stevia and Monk Fruit

Others:
Carob (observe tolerance), vanilla (alcohol free), baking powder (aluminum free), cinnamon, xanthan gum (small quantity).

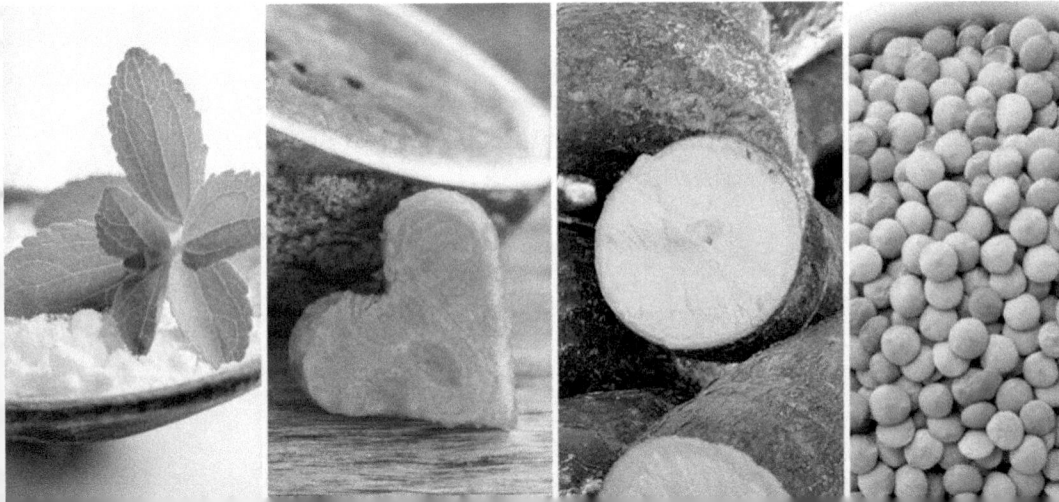

Day 1

» Breakfast: Scrambled eggs with avocado and a portion of baked potatoes or French fries.

» Lunch: Grilled chicken salad with lettuce, shredded carrots, and sesame seeds. Accompanied by 25 to 50 grams of brown rice.

» Dinner: Wild salmon grilled or poached with ghee, asparagus, and green beans as well some cucumbers on the side.

Day 2

» Breakfast: Egg omelet with zucchini and carrots sautéed, and a portion of fried yucca sticks.

» Lunch: Lentils stewed with carrots, peppers, and chicken, served on a portion of quinoa.

» Dinner: Roasted rabbit or pork chops with chayote fried in ghee and a serving of brussels sprouts with avocado.

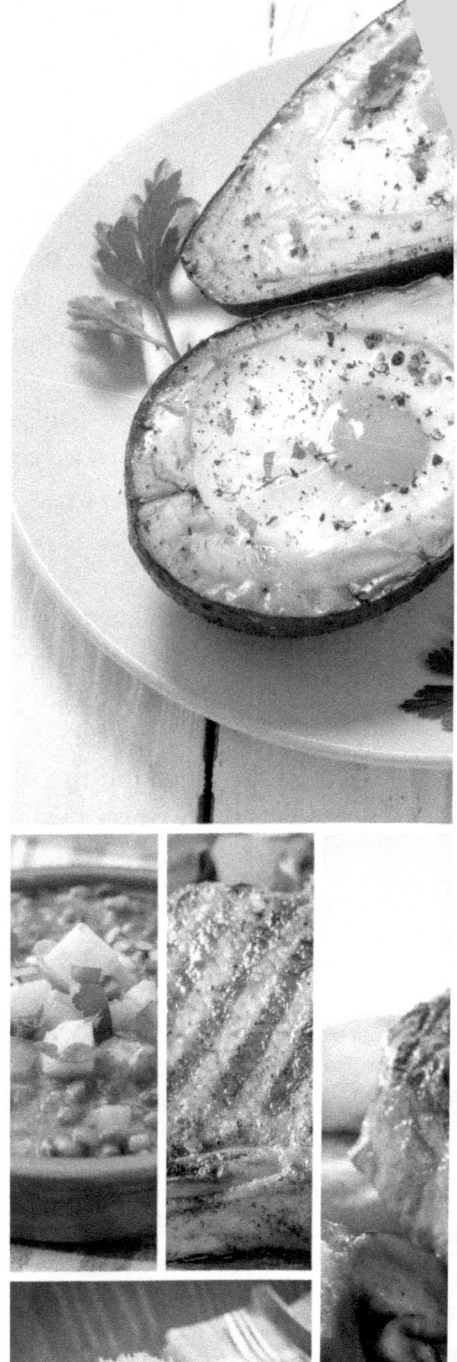

51

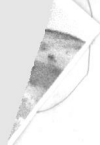

Day 3

» Breakfast: Eggs scrambled in the bacon fat or in ghee with a portion of mashed potatoes and some pork rinds.
» Lunch: Chicken with zucchini fried in ghee with bell peppers with 25 or 50 grams of quinoa.
» Dinner: Grilled wild salmon with asparagus wrapped in bacon and a side of avocado and lettuce salad.

Day 4

» Breakfast: Poached eggs with shredded chicken and a serving of macadamia nuts.
» Lunch: Beans with shredded beef, accompanied by 25 or 50 gr of quinoa or rice and zucchini salad.
» Dinner: Beef filet with ghee with sauteed zucchini and a side salad of cucumbers and carrots.

Day 5

» Breakfast: Scrambled eggs with asparagus, diced peppers, and some chaffles.
» Lunch: Shrimp salad with lettuce, cucumber, carrots, and olive oil. Accompanied by 25 or 50 gr of quinoa or rice
» Dinner: Grilled lamb filet with asparagus and 25 or 50 gr of quinoa or rice.

Day 6

> » Breakfast: Waffles or hotcakes/pancakes, coconut flour and scrambled eggs
> » Lunch: Duck or chicken with asparagus and a portion of mashed potatoes (25 or 50 gr)
> » Dinner: Grilled chicken with asparagus and French fries (25 or 50 gr)

Day 7

> » Breakfast: Egg omelet with pork rinds and a portion of macadamias.
> » Lunch: Grilled wild salmon with a portion of brown rice (25 or 50 gr) and zucchini sautéed with ghee.
> » Dinner: Hamburger with a cloud bread bun with asparagus and some French fries (25 or 50 gr)

SNACKS/SNACKS BETWEEN FOODS CAN BE NUTS, SEEDS, PORK RINDS OR RAW VEGETABLES SUCH AS JICAMA (MEXICAN TURNIP), CUCUMBER, CELERY AND/OR CARROTS.

» We suggest limiting the consumption of fruits, since they are high in fructose, which is sugar. Sugar feeds pathogens as well as causing inflammation in the body. If your child really likes fruits, we recommend consuming between 150 and 200 grams twice a week and they should consume them away from the main meals. One apple or pear is the maximum per day. There are children who eat 5 to 8 pieces of fruit a day, plus juices, etc. It is a big problem when we want to heal the intestine and the person. **You must always be leery of sugar even if it is in a natural form.**

» These meal plans are just an example of how we can combine foods. You can adapt it to your child's individual needs.

Chapter 4
Toxin Moppers, Chelators, CD and Minerals

- Toxin Collectors
- Ultra binder, H7 and PektiClean
- Salt Baths
- CD
- Magnesium
- Potassium

CHAPTER 4

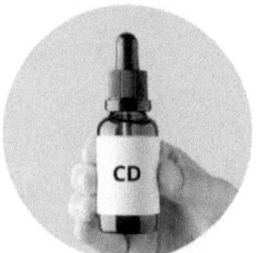

Toxin Moppers, Chelators, CD and Minerals

Dear Parents:

It is vitally important that we understand that each child is unique and may react differently to different foods or supplements. Therefore, I recommend that you start supplementation gradually, starting with one supplement at a time, with a day or 2 in between starting another supplement. As well as adjusting the doses according to your child's individual reaction.

It is extremely important to keep a detailed diary or log in which you note any changes or reactions in your child. This record will help us to evaluate progress and determine if dosage adjustments or protocol modifications are necessary. Keep in mind that this process requires perseverance and patience, since each child may need a different adaptation time.

Each phase in the protocol does not replace the previous one, but rather adds to it. As they progress through the protocol, they will incorporate new stages until they achieve an ATEC (Autism Treatment Evaluation Checklist) score of less than 10, which indicates that the child is recovered. The ATEC of 0 is what we are always looking for. Which indicates that there are no traits left of the autism spectrum.

Communication with Kerri or the support group facilitators is extremely important.

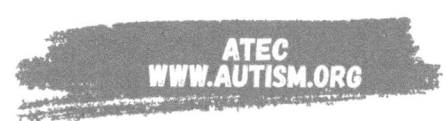

ATEC
WWW.AUTISM.ORG

They will be very helpful in providing personalized guidance and responding to your concerns based on your child's individual needs.

We deeply appreciate your commitment and dedication to caring for your child. By working together, we can advance on the path towards their well-being and full healing.

MY EMAIL IS:
KERRI@KERRIRIVERA.COM

ULTRA BINDER
(Toxin and heavy metal mopper)

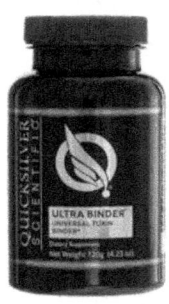

It is a large molecule that stays in and travels through the intestine for the specific purpose of detoxifying it. It contains a complete mix of natural components that effectively bind with various toxins and heavy metals present in our daily lives. This process facilitates a safe and organic detoxification of the intestines. It comes out of the body the next day in the feces.

This formula is especially effective in removing toxic compounds such as heavy metals, pesticides, herbicides, endocrine disruptors, drug residues, food additives, as well as toxins derived from mold/fungus, parasites, and bacteria.

When using Ultrabinder, your stool may take on a blackish or greenish hue, which is a normal due to the ingredients in the Ultra binder.

Dilute in 1 or 2 ounces/30 to 60 ml of water or non-dairy milk and take every night before bed 5 minutes after the last dose of CD.

Weight in pounds	Weight in kg	Dose
25 lb	11 kg	¼ teaspoon
50 lb	22.5 kg	½ teaspoon
75 lb	34 kg	¾ teaspoon
100 pounds and up	45 kg	1 tablespoon

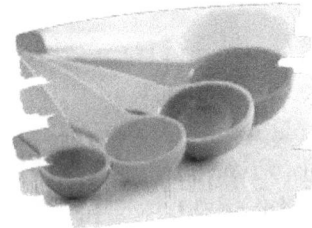

Whenever we talk about teaspoon measurements, we are referring to the number of measuring spoons used in baking or cooking.

FORMULA H-7

The urea cycle is an important process in our body that helps eliminate toxic waste substances from ammonia. Parasites release a lot of ammonia. Our body produces small amounts of ammonia when we digest proteins in food. The function of the urea cycle is to convert ammonia into urea, a less toxic substance that is eliminated through urine.

The liver is the main organ responsible for metabolizing and eliminating ammonia through the urea cycle. The H7 formula contains all the 7 amino acids in the urea cycle that are responsible for eliminating toxic ammonia from the body.

The urea cycle is essential to keeping us healthy and preventing toxic ammonia from building up in our body. High ammonia can affect the brain so much that it can cause behavioral problems, tiredness, and even serious health problems such as seizures/epilepsy and coma. Signs and symptoms of hyperammonemia may include confusion.

IF YOUR CHILD IS TAKING GABA, BOTH SUPPLEMENTS CAN BE GIVEN SIMULTANEOUSLY

SUGGESTED DOSAGE OF H-7 BASED ON WEIGHT

In Pounds	In kg	Dose
Up to 25 lb	Up to 11 kg	1 capsule 2 times a day
26 lb – 50 lb	12 kg–22 kg	2 capsules 2 times a day
51 lb – 75 lb	23 kg–34 kg	3 capsules 2 times a day
76 lb – 100 lb and up	35 kg – 45 kg and up	4 capsules 2 times a day

PEKTICLEAN

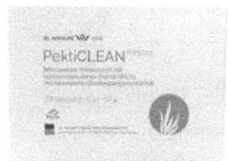

PektiClean ® The import and export of molecules into and out of the cell is carried out through the plasma membrane.

However, not all molecules can easily cross this barrier. The apple pectin molecule, for example, cannot penetrate the cell due to its size.

The PektiClean® molecule, on the other hand, can freely penetrate the cell membrane and bind contaminants directly there. PektiClean® has a low molecular content of up to 60%, is negatively charged and unsaturated. This creates a strong attraction towards positively charged particles such as oxides or toxins. Therefore, the low molecular weight portion of PektiClean® combines with toxins to produce a saturated compound. The saturated compound thus formed is excreted through the liver and kidneys. There is nothing else like it on the market. It takes out toxins and heavy metals from the whole body including the brain.

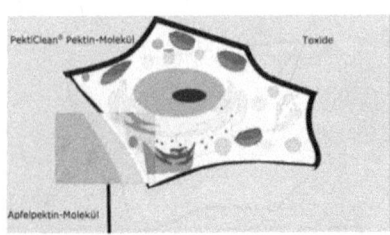 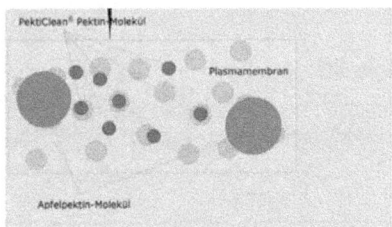

SUGGESTED USE

Mix the recommended dose of Pekticlean in 2 ounces/60ml of warm water or drink as a tea. You cannot eat anything one hour before or half an hour after taking Pekticlean. This supplement can be taken once or twice a day, or when the child is having a healing crisis, such as Herxheimer's symptoms.

In Pounds	In kg	Dose
25 lb	11 kg	¼ of envelope
50 lb	22 kg	½ of envelope
100 lb	45 kg	1 envelope

SALT BATHS

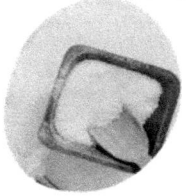 If you do not have access to any of the toxin collectors (Ultra binder, H-7, Pekticlean) salt baths can help mitigate toxins a little, due to the osmosis effect it causes in the body.

When you immerse yourself in a bath of highly salty water, your skin acts as a semi-permeable barrier. The salt water in the bathtub has a higher concentration of salt compared to the cells in your body. Due to this difference in concentration, the process of osmosis occurs, water begins to enter your skin and leave your cells due to the difference in concentration. This can have several beneficial effects like how to help eliminate toxins and waste accumulated in the body by extracting them through the skin.

INSTRUCTIONS FOR SALT BATHS

» 4 kg of cheap salt (You can use the cheapest table salt you can find on the market)
» Fill the bathtub with warm to hot water at what would be considered a comfortable temperature. Make sure the water covers the entire body when you get in the tub (from the neck down).
» Add the salt to the water, stirring the water with your hand to help dissolve the salt.
» If you want to add a relaxing aroma, you can add a few drops of lavender essential oil, chamomile, or any other essential oil. Make sure the essential oil is formulated for use in baths. (Optional)
» Once the tub is full and the salt has dissolved, soak in the water and relax for 20 to 40 minutes or more. There is no time limit to be there.

» After finishing the bath, rinse your body with enough water to remove the salt and drink enough water to keep your body hydrated, as salt baths can dehydrate the skin. You can apply black seed oil to your skin afterwards for hydration especially if there is any drying of the skin from the baths.

» Remember that if you have any irritation or open wound on your skin, you should not take the salt bath because it will irritate the skin even more.

What is CD?

Chlorine Dioxide (CD) is a pro-oxidant, considered a biocidal agent due to its ability to reduce the toxic load of pathogens such as bacteria, viruses, parasites, and fungi through an oxidation process when it comes into contact with them. CD kills pathogens by oxidation and neutralizes heavy metals. CD is a gas and will travel freely throughout the body. It is a selective killer. It will only kill pathogens. CD is a positively charged molecule and is repelled by healthy cells and friendly flora. CD does no harm to the body. CD is attracted to the negatively charged pathogens and is destroyed in the process of killing pathogens. CD is active in the body for approximately 45 minutes.

HOW IS CD MADE?

The most common and easiest method is to mix sodium chlorite (NaClO2) and the activator HCl 4%. When these two substances react together, they release chlorine dioxide (CD) gas.

This gas molecule is very small and simple, containing one chlorine atom (Cl) and two oxygen atoms (O2). It is extremely soluble in water and does not create chemical bonds. This means that the gas can completely dissolve in water. Thanks to this property, it can be used to purify water safely and effectively, while completely inactivating viruses, bacteria, fungi and some types of small parasites. There is no residue, it does not accumulate in the body, and you can take it every day of your life.

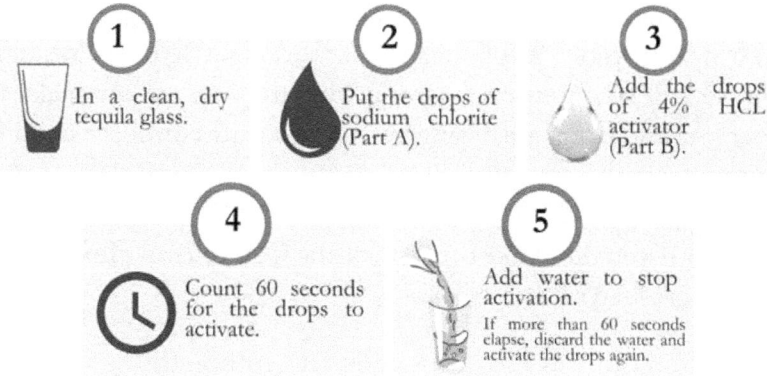

1. In a clean, dry tequila glass.

2. Put the drops of sodium chlorite (Part A).

3. Add the drops of 4% HCL activator (Part B).

4. Count 60 seconds for the drops to activate.

5. Add water to stop activation.
If more than 60 seconds elapse, discard the water and activate the drops again.

It is important to note that when we talk about CD drops, we are referring to activated drops.

For every drop of sodium chlorite, you will need the same number of drops of the 4% HCl activator. The ratio should be 1:1. For example, if you activate 1 drop of CD, you must place 1 drop of sodium chlorite and 1 drop of the 4% HCl activator in the glass. Wait 45 to 60 seconds for it to activate. Once that time has passed, add water to stop the activation and add to a bottle of water.

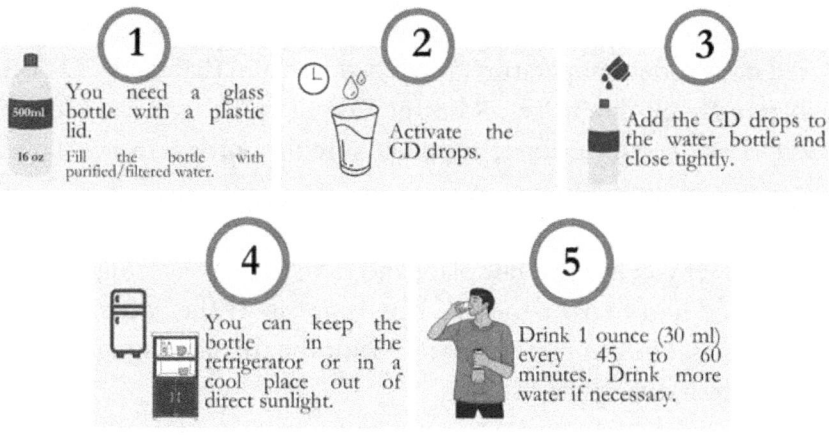

1. You need a glass bottle with a plastic lid. Fill the bottle with purified/filtered water.

2. Activate the CD drops.

3. Add the CD drops to the water bottle and close tightly.

4. You can keep the bottle in the refrigerator or in a cool place out of direct sunlight.

5. Drink 1 ounce (30 ml) every 45 to 60 minutes. Drink more water if necessary.

» Take 30ml/1oz from the 500ml/16oz bottle every 45 minutes throughout the day starting the moment you wake up till you go to bed. If possible, it is better to get more than 16 doses in a day. If the 500ml/16oz bottle runs out during the day, you can make another one and continue dosing every 45 minutes until the child falls asleep at night.

» If you don't like the taste of the CD, you can dilute the shot with more water if necessary.

» You can also add drops of SweetLeaf brand stevia to the additional water that you will use to transfer the flavor of the CD. We have tested many brands of stevia, including natural and organic stevia, and they all cut the potency of CD. The only one that maintained the potency of the CD was SweetLeaf's stevia.

» If you cannot finish the bottle of CD for the day, it is not necessary to discard the remaining doses in the bottle, as long as the bottle has a tightly closed lid it will be fine to use the next day. The CD bottle maintains its potential for up to 72 hours. It can be stored in the refrigerator overnight.

» You can keep the bottle with the day's CD doses refrigerated or at room temperature. Most people claim that cold CD tastes better. If you don't like cold drinks, don't worry, you can keep the CD at room temperature, just make sure the bottle is in a cool place and out of sunlight.

» If you live in a hot place and have to be away from home, it is a good idea to use a thermal bag to transport the bottle with the CD doses, You can place ice packs inside the thermal bag to ensure it stays fresh during your outing.

CALCULATING CD DOSES

There is no maximum number of doses. CD is taken as tolerated. I have seen people improve with 24 drops and others who reach 80 drops without any problem. It all depends on the tolerance of each person. We work up slowly. Increasing by 1 drop per day. The vast majority of people tolerate drops based on their weight. I have a list of drops by weight here.

If your child presents symptoms such as: nausea, tiredness, or lack of appetite, this means that his/her body is releasing toxins rapidly. In this case, you should go slower and increase the drops every 3 or 4 days.

Although there is a table with suggested doses based on weight, it is always best to adjust the dose according to each person's tolerance. For example, if the recommended dose for your child to take is 20 drops based on their weight, but at drop number 17 they start to feel nauseous or lose their appetite, you need to go back to drop 16 or the drop where they were fine and stay there, because that's the dose that their body tolerates.

The important thing is to maintain the CD frequency in the body. So the pathogens cannot gain strength or continue to multiply. We have seen cases where they focus on reaching the dose according to weight, but then they must stop because of nausea and that is precisely what we should avoid. The most important thing is the frequency of the dosing of CD. That is, 16 doses or more a day is what matters. The number of drops that are tolerated is what is important about the drops. There should never be less than 16 doses of CD a day. We need to keep pressure on the pathogens so that they cannot continue to multiply and divide. We need to have more hours of killing pathogens then they must multiply.

Weight in kg	Suggested dose	Weight in kg	Suggested dose
11	16 drops	31	38 drops
12	16 drops	32	38 drops
13	18 drops	33	38 drops
14	20 drops	34	40 drops
15	20 drops	35	40 drops
16	22 drops	36	40 drops
17	22 drops	37	42 drops
18	24 drops	38	42 drops
19	26 drops	39	42 drops
20	28 drops	40	44 drops
21	30 drops	41	44 drops
22	30 drops	42	44 drops
23	32 drops	43	46 drops
24	32 drops	44	46 drops
25	34 drops	45	46 drops
26	34 drops	46	48 drops
27	34 drops	47	48 drops
28	36 drops	48	48 drops
29	36 drops	49	50 drops
30	36 drops	50	50 drops

» This table guides you and shows you the suggested dose according to your child's weight.

» **Adjust the dose according to your tolerance:** Although the dosage is based on weight, it is best to adapt the dosage according to your child's tolerance.

» **Dilute in 16 ounces/500ml of water:** Mix the suggested dose in a 16-ounce/500ml glass bottle of water. If you feel that the taste is too strong, you should add the dose of CD to additional water before drinking the dose. You can add the 1oz/30ml dose to as much water as to make it palatable.

» **Dosing frequency:** Administer one dose of CD every 45 minutes from the time they wake up till they go to bed.

CD DOSE CONTROL

NAME:
ATEC:
DATE:

DOSE	TIME	COMMENTS
💧 1	🕐	💬
💧 2	🕐	💬
💧 3	🕐	💬
💧 4	🕐	💬
💧 5	🕐	💬
💧 6	🕐	💬
💧 7	🕐	💬
💧 8	🕐	💬
💧 9	🕐	💬
💧 10	🕐	💬
💧 11	🕐	💬
💧 12	🕐	💬
💧 13	🕐	💬
💧 14	🕐	💬
💧 15	🕐	💬
💧 16	🕐	💬

NOTES:

EVERY SMALL STEP TOWARD PROGRESS IS A GREAT ACHIEVEMENT FOR YOUR CHILD AND FOR YOU.

Suggestions for doing the enema

Gather the necessary supplies: Enema bag, syringes with catheters or enema pump, disposable towel or pad, water-soluble lubricant like silver gel, disposable gloves, and toilet paper.

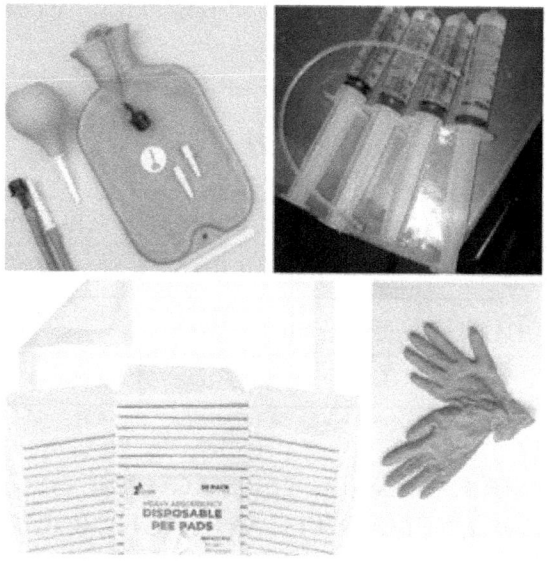

Find a comfortable, private spot in the bathroom, near a surface where you can lie down, and use a disposable cover, towel, or pad.

Warm the filtered water to body temperature (approximately 37°C). Make sure the water is not hot. You can test the temperature with the back of your hand to make sure it is comfortable. The person giving the enema to another person should wear disposable gloves.

Position the person so that the water goes in more quickly. It is important that we are in the position of elbows and knees on the floor. You must think about the gravity of the earth.

Apply water-soluble lubricant like silver gel to the catheter that goes into the body or coconut oil. Also put lubricant on the rectum as well.

Carefully insert the tip of the probe or catheter into the rectum, making sure not to force it and keeping it pointed toward the belly button. Normally, we put half of the catheter into the body. So, it doesn't come out during the enema process. We do the enema quickly in seconds not minutes.

Administer the solution as quickly as possible or according to your child's pace.

DOSAGE FOR ENEMA

Age	Water	CD drops
Children – up to 9 years	1 liter	10
10 to 15 years	2 liters	20
Adults	3 liters	30

CLEANING AFTER EACH USE OF
THE ENEMA WITH SYRINGE OR BAG

» Completely empty the enema bag or syringes and rinse them with hot water.

» Make sure to clean all parts and rinse them properly, then spray all parts with alcohol (use a spray bottle).

» If necessary, disassemble the equipment for a more complete cleaning.

» Allow all parts to dry completely before storing. You can place them in a clean, well-ventilated area or use a clean towel to dry them.

CLEANING AFTER EACH USE
WITH ENEMA PUMP

» Completely empty the pump.

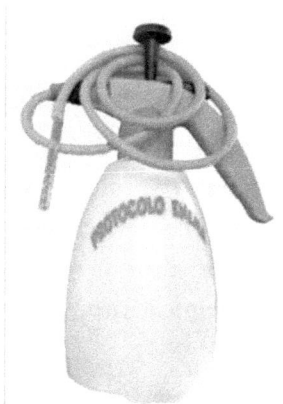

» Thoroughly wash the acrylic tip with hot water to ensure complete cleaning and remove any traces of feces.

» Prepare a disinfectant solution with CD: with 20 drops of CD per 30ml/1oz of water.

» Place the CD disinfectant solution into a spray bottle.

» Allow the CD disinfectant solution to run through the entire hose, including the acrylic tip.

» Let the water drain completely from the pump.

» Store the pump in a cabinet in your bathroom, making sure it is dry and ready for next use.

» There is no need to disassemble the entire equipment, as the pump is hermetically sealed and never comes into contact with feces or other contaminants. This process guarantees effective and safe disinfection for next use.

Frequently asked questions about CD

Is CD chlorine like in is used in pools?

NO! As we learned in high school chemistry classes, combining two compounds can generate a new substance that does not look like its predecessors. An example of chlorine is the mixture of two parts hydrogen gas with one part oxygen, which creates liquid water. We must keep in mind that, although chlorine and chlorine dioxide share the same word, their chemical properties are completely different and should not be confused.

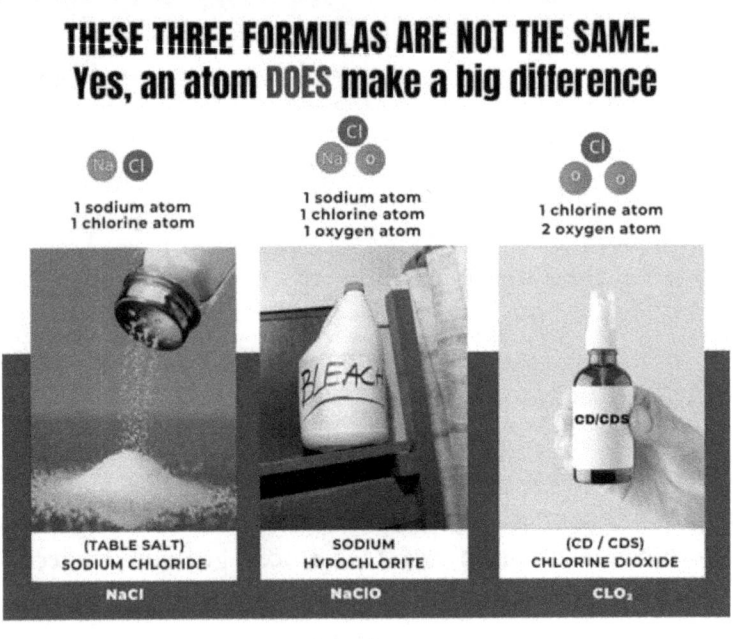

THESE THREE FORMULAS ARE NOT THE SAME.
Yes, an atom DOES make a big difference

1 sodium atom
1 chlorine atom

1 sodium atom
1 chlorine atom
1 oxygen atom

1 chlorine atom
2 oxygen atom

(TABLE SALT)
SODIUM CHLORIDE
$NaCl$

SODIUM
HYPOCHLORITE
$NaClO$

(CD / CDS)
CHLORINE DIOXIDE
ClO_2

KERRI RIVERA

For more information click here:
https://www.scotmas.com/chlorine-dioxide/why-is-clo2-different-to-chlorine.aspx?locale=enom/chlorine-dioxide/why-is-clo2-different-to-chlorine.aspx?locale=en

Does CD cause oxidative stress?

NO! CD does not cause oxidative stress, oxidative stress is caused when there are an excess of pathogens in the body.

When the immune system is under excessive load from pathogens, such as bacteria, parasites or other microorganisms, a chronic inflammatory response can occur. During this response, immune cells release free radicals and other reactive oxygen species to attempt to eliminate invading pathogens. However, if the pathogen load is too high or the inflammatory response becomes chronic, there may be excessive accumulation of free radicals.

Excess pathogens can trigger a chronic inflammatory response and, consequently, cause oxidative stress in the body. It is essential to lower the toxic load to reduce oxidative stress. Eliminating pathogens is key to reducing the overall body inflammation and burden of oxidative stress due to excess pathogens.

Does CD damage the good intestinal flora?

No, CD does not harm the good gut flora, the beneficial bacteria in the gut have a negative (-) charge, which allows them to repel each other and distribute themselves evenly.

CD has a negative (-) charge just like the good gut flora and (-) and (-) repel each other. Pathogens have a positive (+) charge. In contrast, opposite charges attract. In other words, negative (-) and positive (+) charges have a mutual attraction, just as when you bring the negative and positive poles of two magnets closer together.

Does CD damage good intestinal flora?

NO! CD does not damage the friendly (beneficial) gut flora of the intestine. The beneficial bacteria in the intestine have a positive charge (+), which allows them to repel each other and distribute themselves in a balanced way.

CD has a positive charge (+) just like the beneficial gut flora of the intestine and + and + repel each other. Pathogens have a negative (-) charge so the CD will be drawn to the pathogen. CD is a selective killer. It does not kill indiscriminately. CD will only kill pathogens never damaging the good, healthy, friendly, beneficial gut flora. In contrast, opposite charges attract. That is, negative (-) and positive (+) charges have a mutual attraction, just like when you bring the negative and positive poles of two magnets closer together.

In conclusion, positive charges (+) repel beneficial bacteria and opposite charges like positive and negative attract each other. These interactions are essential for maintaining a healthy balance of bacteria in the intestine.

Does CD interfere with other medications?

No, CD does not interfere with any medications. A separation in delivery time is not necessary.

Is it true that lemon (citrus) negates the power of the CD?
Yes, lemon (all citrus), vitamin C and any other antioxidant supplements counteract the effect of the CD.

I started taking CD and I feel sick, why is this?

When we take CD, antifungals, antibiotics, anthelmintics to combat pathogens and parasites, sometimes a Herxheimer (healing crisis) may occur. This is due to the destruction of the pathogens which release toxicity in our body.

These symptoms are known as Herxheimer's reaction and usually occur in the form of nausea, tiredness, diarrhea, joint pain, headache, or a worsening of any of the many symptoms that pathogens can produce. Although it may be uncomfortable, a Herxheimer reaction is generally a sign that treatment is working and toxins are being eliminated from the body. It's a good time to use Pekticlean to mop up those toxins in the body.

My child suffers from constipation. Can I start enemas before reaching the dosage that corresponds to your weight?

Anyone suffering from constipation needs enemas immediately. It is important to encourage bowel movements in any detox protocol. When there is constipation, we do not wait for the maximum dose to start enemas. In reality, it is best to start enemas ASAP. The enema helps to detoxify the liver. That is the principle reason for the enema to begin with. And of course, the CD in the water of the enema helps to destroy biofilm in the gut which provides home to countless pathogens and heavy metals.

Magnesium

Magnesium is essential for the optimal chemical functioning of the human body, participating in metabolic reactions, nucleic acid synthesis, muscle contraction, electrolyte balance, glucose regulation, anti-inflammatory effects, antioxidant protection and health of the nervous system.

There are different forms of magnesium, such as magnesium citrate, magnesium threonate, magnesium glycinate, magnesium malate, among others. Each form has different characteristics and bioavailability, meaning they are absorbed and used differently by the body. Magnesium citrate and magnesium glycinate usually have better absorption and are recommended in cases of autism.

Magnesium citrate:

Magnesium citrate is considered to be a highly bioavailable form of magnesium, meaning it is easily absorbed into the body. This allows better utilization of magnesium by cells and tissue of the body.

It is of great help in cases of constipation because it helps relax the muscles of the intestine by drawing water into the intestine, which increases the water content in the stool. This helps soften the stool and makes it easier to pass through the intestine.

Magnesium Citrate Dosage:

Start with one capsule, each day increase one more capsule until mild diarrhea occurs. If mild diarrhea occurs after 3 capsules, the next day return to two capsules and stay there. You can take it with every meal. Take as much as needed to move the bowels at least 1 time a day.

We have seen cases that require 4 or 6 magnesium capsules several times a day with each meal and diarrhea never appears. Magnesium with each meal is a good way to administer it.

Magnesium citrate dosage depends on each person. When someone suffers from constipation, the amount of magnesium citrate increases until they have 1 to 3 doses a day with meals. It is important to have a bowel movement 1 to 3 times a day.

Magnesium Glycinate:

It is characterized by its high bioavailability and tolerability. In cases where someone has with soft stools or diarrhea, magnesium glycinate is undoubtedly the best option.

Magnesium Glycinate Dosage:

One of the benefits of this form of magnesium is that it promotes restful sleep. I like to divide the dose of magnesium with each meal. It helps to keep the nervous system calm. This helps with focus, language and behaviors. If your child takes GABA you can give both supplements together. Children 300 to 600 mg – Adults 600 to 1000 mg. These doses can be much higher. It all depends on how the person responds. Magnesium can help all of us rest better in the evenings. Not just our children.

Potassium Citrate

Potassium is very important for the body to function normally. It is a type of electrolyte. It helps nerve function and muscle contraction and keeps your heart rate constant. It also allows nutrients to flow to the cells and waste to be expelled from them. **LOW LEVELS OF POTASSIUM CAN CAUSE MUSCLE CRAMPING, WEAKNESS, FATIGUE ETC.**

SUGGESTED DOSAGE OF POTASSIUM CITRATE

In pounds	In kg	Dose
25 lb – 99 lb	11 kg–44 kg	50 mg with food and magnessium
100 lb and up	45 kg and up	100 mg with food and magnessium

Chapter 5
Basic Supplements

- Humic/Fulvic
- Chondroitin sulfate/oleic acid/D
- Structured Silver
- Black Seed Oil
- Super Enzymes
- Betaine HCl

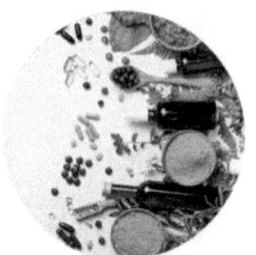

Basic Supplements

Humic/Fulvic

Humic/Fulvic is a combination of humic and fulvic acids, organic nutrients extracted from virgin and ancient soils. These compounds contain a diversity of essential nutrients, including amino acids, minerals, nucleic acids and phytochemical compounds. It has been used in Ayurvedic medicine and has been shown to have beneficial health properties by improving nutrient absorption, balancing the gut microbiome, supporting the immune system, and facilitating the elimination of toxins from the body. It crosses the blood-brain barrier and removes heavy metals from the brain, among other benefits.

BENEFITS OF HUMIC/FULVIC

- » Improves nutrient absorption at the cellular level.
- » Balances the intestinal microbiome.
- » Increases blood oxygenation.
- » Support the immune system.
- » Reduces inflammation.
- » Facilitates the elimination of toxins from the body.
- » Crosses the blood-brain barrier and removes heavy metals from the brain.
- » Seals leaky gut.
- » Regulates the bioavailability of iron, calcium, magnesium and copper.

» Used in Ayurvedic medicine to treat digestive and immune system diseases.
» Improves circulation and immunity.
» Reduces pain.
» Reduces susceptibility to infections, including SIBO, bacterial infections and colds.
» Improves digestion and absorption of nutrients.
» Provides electrolytes and trace elements for proper metabolic functions.
» Helps prevent free radicals that can cause cognitive disorders such as Alzheimer's.
» Relieves constipation, bloating, diarrhea and food sensitivities.
» It has neuroprotective and chelating properties.
» Binds and breaks down toxins in the body.
» Repairs and protects the skin.
» It contributes to the longevity of cells in the brain, heart, muscles and digestive tract.
» Benefits in conditions such as gastritis, diarrhea, stomach ulcers, colitis and diabetes.
» Stimulates bone growth.
» Improves sleep quality and recovery after training.
» It contributes to the rewiring of the brain and the elimination of negative neurons.
» It has antibiotic properties
» Optimizes mitochondrial functions.
» Facilitates the absorption of nutrients and detoxifies the body.
» Silica increases collagen synthesis.
» It can act as a prebiotic and probiotic.

Properties:

  » Antioxidant
  » Antimicrobial
  » Antifungal
  » Antiviral
  » Anti-inflammatory
  » Anti-allergy
  » Antimutagenic
  » Antibiotic
  » Antispasmodic

SUGGESTED USE

  » Children: 13 drops, 3 times a day.
  » Young people and adults: 25 drops, 3 times a day.
  » You can take Humic/Fulvic with and without food.
  » For easy use, dilute it in water, soup/broth or your favorite beverage.
  » You can also add the drops directly to your food.
  » Humic/Fulvic is tasteless, odorless, does not affect the effectiveness of other supplements or medications, and does not require refrigeration.

IT HAS BEEN DEMONSTRATED TO POSSESS HEALTH-ENHANCING PROPERTIES, IMPROVING NUTRIENT ABSORPTION, BALANCING THE INTESTINAL MICROBIOME, SUPPORTING THE IMMUNE SYSTEM, AND FACILITATING THE ELIMINATION OF TOXINS FROM THE BODY.

Seawater (ocean water) vs. Humic/fulvic

Why is HUMIC/FULVIC better than Sea water (ocean water)?

What is the difference between seawater and HUMIC/FULVIC as a source of minerals and support for general health?

The question deserves an in-depth answer. Let's start by looking at the claims made about seawater and then compare them to what is known about HUMIC/FULVIC.

There is extensive scientific research examining the properties of HUMIC/FULVIC in relation to both soil health and human health. In this section I will seek to summarize this research. Let's assume that both seawater and HUMIC/FULVIC have been obtained from the best available sources, so the comparison will be of the intrinsic values of each rather than their sources. Since the oceans can be contaminated. Humic/Fulvic comes from deep in the earth and is not possible to be adulterated by a toxic world.

In the case of seawater, it has been extracted from the depths of a vortex, the life engine of the ocean. Most people selling ocean water are not getting it from the vortex FYI. Quinton is likely the only one that sells seawater getting it from the vortex. Humic/Fulvic have been drawn from deep within a vein that has taken hundreds of thousands, if not millions of years to develop.

HUMIC/FULVIC

The question deserves an in-depth answer. Let's start by looking at the claims made about seawater and then compare them to what is known about HUMIC/FULVIC.

There is extensive scientific research examining the properties of HUMIC/FULVIC in relation to both soil health and human health.

In this section I will seek to summarize this research. Let's assume that both seawater and HUMIC/FULVIC have been obtained from the best available sources, so the comparison will be of the intrinsic values of each rather than their sources. Since the oceans can be contaminated. Humic/Fulvic comes from deep in the earth and is not possible to be adulterated by a toxic world.

In the case of seawater, it has been extracted from the depths of a vortex, the life engine of the ocean. Most people selling ocean water are not getting it from the vortex FYI. Quinton is likely the only one that sells seawater getting it from the vortex. Humic/Fulvic have been drawn from deep within a vein that has taken hundreds of thousands, if not millions of years to develop.

SEA WATER VS. HUMIC/FULVIC

HUMIC/FULVIC act as carrier molecules or chelating agents for smaller, more bioactive compounds. (Schepetkin et al., 2002, citing Ghosal et al., 1991; Meena, 2010, citing Shenyuan et al., 1993; Pant et al., 2012)

HUMIC/FULVIC is not a good source of iodine. Research clearly shows that HUMIC/FULVIC provides everything AND MORE that seawater provides except iodine, and in fact, they provide these properties in a much more potent and bioavailable way. But the differences between the two are not just ones of degree. Seawater has much more sodium than HUMIC/FULVIC, which is not good. In fact, soil high in sodium prevents or even eliminates the ability of plants to grow. Interestingly, HUMIC/FULVIC can be used to rehabilitate high sodium soils and make them fertile again. (Pettit, 2004) HUMIC/FULVIC are not only used to restore saline soils but are also used to mitigate all types of toxic pollution. (Pandey et al, 2000; Kochany et al., 2001; Burlakovs et al., 2013)

Why is this important? Because the same principle that allows HUMIC/FULVIC to rehabilitate contaminated soil also works inside the human body with regards to gut flora. HUMIC/FULVIC is a natural chelator that not only neutralizes toxins, but also helps eliminate them from the tissues and brain. (Schepetkin et al., 2002, citing Schnitzer and Khan, 1972)

Seawater does not have this capacity. Even more importantly, HUMIC/FULVIC is a better source of minerals. HUMIC/FULVIC has 75+ minerals. Seawater only has 45 minerals and several of these are heavy metals. If both provide numerous minerals, trace elements and electrolytes, how can HUMIC/FULVIC be better? Simply put, HUMIC/FULVIC, especially HUMIC/FULVIC, acts as a transport to carry minerals into the cells and seawater cannot do that. Seawater can provide minerals to the body, but it cannot get them into the cells like HUMIC/FULVIC does. The body can use the minerals in seawater, but the energy expended to move them into the cells is much greater than when HUMIC/FULVIC is present to move the minerals into the cells. (Schepetkin et al., 2002, citing Schnitzer and Khan, 1972) HUMIC/FULVIC can penetrate the cell better than any other substance in nature.

The combination of chelating properties and cell penetrating properties found in HUMIC/FULVIC makes them far superior to seawater and to any other mineral supplement. Yes, seawater has iodine, but when weighed in comparison, the most versatile product becomes clear, HUMIC/FULVIC wins bar none. Remember that capsules with minerals in them are not the best way to get multiminerals. You want a liquid, bioavailable one as is HUMIC/FULVIC. There is just no comparison to anything else on the market. At the end of the day, the goal is to heal the body as fast as possible. This is the best way that I have seen in 20 years of testing and using supplements.

Condroitin Sulfate/Oleic Acid/D

Is a macrophage activator and a nagalase reducer. Macrophages are cells of the immune system that play a fundamental role in defending the body against infections and diseases. They are part of the mononuclear phagocytic system and are present in different tissues of the body.

Macrophages are like "PAC-MAN" that go through the body engulfing pathogens such as bacteria, fungi, viruses, parasites, and tumors. Macrophages also go after viruses associated with influenza, the common cold, and measles. Our advanced formula activates these macrophages and supports control of pathogens that cause disease and inflammation. Email for links. We are very censored.

It supports the immune system, bone health, and reduces the toxic load in the body. We have observed substantial improvements in; behavior, language, socialization as well as cognition. There have been studies on this product as a registered trademark.

https://www.researchgate.net/publication/330920601_Vaccines_Autism_and_RerumR

SUGGESTED USE

» Day 1: Start with one dropper, 6 times a day, with or without food. You can mix it with a little water, non-dairy milk or administer it directly into your mouth.

» Day 2: Increase to two droppers, 6 times a day. Every day for 6 days we went up a drip 6 times a day.

» Watch how your child reacts. If you notice improvement, continue increasing one more dropper, 6 times a day, until you reach 6 droppers, 6 times a day.

» If on day 6 you don't see any improvement, reduce the dose to one dropper, 6 times a day, and stay there.

» It is important to keep the bottle of "Chondroitin Sulfate/ Oleic Acid/D" refrigerated once it has been opened.

» It can be given at the same time as black seed oil and humic/ fulvic with meals and without.

Black Seed Oil

Black seed oil, also known as black cumin oil or Nigella sativa oil, is extracted from the seeds of the Nigella sativa plant, native to Southwest Asia. It has been used throughout history for medicinal and culinary purposes in various cultures, dating back more than 2000 years, as evidenced by the time of King Tutankhamun, and has maintained its prominence, especially among the Muslim community since the year 600.

This oil is known for its medicinal properties due to its composition rich in essential fatty acids, antioxidants and beneficial substances such as thymoquinone.

Thymoquinone, noted for its multiple benefits, not only supports cellular cleansing and intestinal health, but also possesses anti-inflammatory, antifungal, antibacterial and anthelmintic properties. This substance has proven effective in the treatment of conditions such as encephalomyelitis, diabetes and asthma, while helping to prevent the formation of cancer cells. Its key role lies in its ability to scavenge superoxide radicals, which helps keep essential antioxidant enzymes such as glutathione peroxidase and glutathione-S-transferase, crucial for cleansing and defending the body, active.

1. Promotes heart health
2. Fights fungal infections
3. Reduces allergies and sinus infections.
4. Good for the skin
5. Treatment of skin cancer
6. Acne remedy
7. Eliminator of infections
8. Fertility potency
9. Good for hair
10. Reduces flu and fevers
11. Kills boils or carbuncles.
12. Treats coughs and asthma
13. BSO for diarrhea
14. Reduces Arterial Hypertension
15. Eliminates Insomnia
16. Prevents cramps and muscle spasms.
17. Relieves nausea and stomach discomfort.
18. Treats toothaches
19. Kills the cells of the lucemia
20. Inhibits breast cancer
21. Suppresses and kills cancer of the prostate and colon.
22. Cures syphilis
23. Treats eczema
24. Helps to lose weight
25. Prevents diabetes
26. BSO for convulsions and epilepsy
27. Tonsil Inflammation Relief
28. MRSA (Staphylococcus) Infection
29. Combats addiction to opiates.
30. BSO for scars
31. Suppresses Cervical Cancer
32. Prevents radiation damage
33. Prevents and cures lead intoxication.

34. Improves beard growth
35. BSO for bee stings
36. Helps with chest congestion
37. Treats earaches
38. Effective for eye infections
39. Cures facial paralysis
40. Cures nasal congestion
41. Eliminates gallstones
42. Suppresses hepatic calculi
43. Helps with gas
44. Treats hemorrhoids
45. Relieves headaches and migraines.
46. Strengthens the immune system
47. Helps in lactation
48. Improves memory and fights dementia.
49. Treats moles
50. Relieves insect bites
51. Cures peeling lips
52. Relieves constipation
53. Relieves back and muscle pain
54. Cures rheumatic pains
55. Helps with the stomach
56. Relieves gum infections
57. Suppresses bladder infections
58. Improves dry mouth
59. Treats nosebleeds
60. Rejuvenates burns
61. Combats dandruff
62. Treats joint pain
63. Prevents kidney damage due to diabetes.
64. Regulates menstrual cycles
65. BSO for pregnancy
66. Relieves arthritis
67. Treats ulcers
68. Reduces the need to take painkillers
69. Eliminates the cancerous cells of the brain

70. Decreases anxiety
71. Helps against depression
72. Eliminates dizziness
73. Treats heartburn
74. Relieves stress
75. Prevents and treats alzeihmers
76. Treats meningitis
77. Promotes the health of the kidneys
78. Improves sperm count.
79. Promotes healthy growth of bone marrow.
80. Treats HIV
81. Relieves colic
82. Suppresses bronchitis
83. Repairs prostate problems
84. Improves mood
85. Eliminates chronic fatigue
86. Stimulates urine production
87. Protects against damage caused by heart attack.
88. It helps with morphine addiction.
89. Prevents anemia
90. It protects the brain from Parkinson's disease.
91. Cleans parasites
92. Treats obesity
93. Eliminates cancerous cells in the mouth.
94. Suppresses the growth of liver cancer
95. It favors the health and the functioning of the liver
96. Remedies pancreatic cancer
97. Treats lymphoma
98. Detoxifies the body
99. Treats bone cancer
100. Cleans pores in depth
101. Treats escitsofrenia

» Up to 25 lb (Up to 11 kg)
Dosage: 3 ml, 3 times daily with food.

» 26 lb - 50 lb (12 kg - 22 kg)
Dosage: 7 ml, 3 times daily with food.

» 51 lb - 75 lb (23 kg - 34 kg)
Dose: 10 ml, 3 times daily with food.

» 76 lb - 100 lb and up (35 kg - 45 kg and up)
Dosage: 15 ml, 3 times daily with food.

OIL PULLING AND BLACK SEED OIL

"Oil Pulling" is an ancient therapeutic practice originating in India, integrated in the Ayurvedic healing system. The indication that it is doing its cleaning job well is when the oil becomes milky.

The optimal time to perform oil pulling is in the morning, especially upon waking up. If you choose to do it twice a day, it is advisable to wait at least 4 hours after eating. You can drink liquids up to 1 hour before oil pulling.

To start, it is suggested to use 1 teaspoon of black seed oil and gradually increase to 1 tablespoon. Although it is advised to keep the oil in your mouth for at least 10 minutes, it is okay to start with 5 minutes and gradually increase over time.

Some people choose to perform this practice while showering to save time in the morning. However, it is crucial to be careful not to swallow the oil once it has become milky, as it contains bacteria and living organisms that could be harmful.

It is necessary to spit it out to avoid ingesting these substances that have just been eliminated from the body.

Structured Silver with Balanced pH

Promotes a balance in intestinal health, effectively eliminating unwanted pathogens through the ionization process. It is alkaline and does not damage the intestinal flora. 99% of the structured silver leaves the body in 24 hours. None of the other silvers have this ability. It is important that one understands that it IS NOT colloidal silver nor ionic silver of the past. Please never use colloidal nor ionic silver orally. This structured silver is the avant-garde of silvers.

WHY WOULD YOU CHOOSE STRUCTURED SILVER AS A SOLUTION?

Other silver products on the market are acidic and do not work with the body's immune system. The structured silver does not accumulate in the body, nor does it metabolize in the body. Meaning it stays the same from mouth to bladder and colon. It has been formulated to be efficient in its purpose and 99% will be gone in under 24 hours.

FEATURES AND BENEFITS:

- » pH balanced to work in harmony with the body.
- » Free of harmful ingredients and preservatives.
- » Safe to be ingested and used for oral care.

OPTION 1:

Add the structured silver to the water thermos (plastic BPA free) your child will take to school. Don't worry, there is no risk of overdose, your child can consume structured silver water in small or large sips and gulps during the time they are at school.

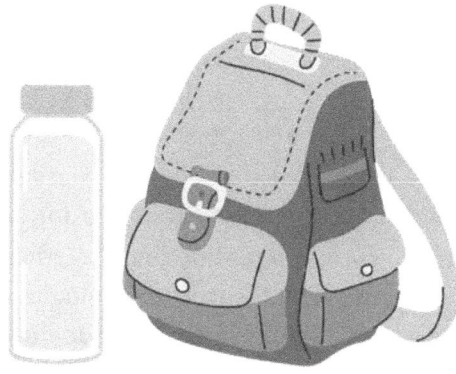

It is important that the thermos is made of plastic (PBA free) or glass, not stainless steel.

Dose for option 1:
> » Children between 2 and 5 years: 40 ml of structured silver.
> » People from 6 years and older: 60 ml of structured silver.

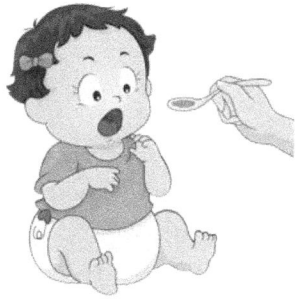

OPTION 2:

Administer structured silver (undiluted) directly into your child's mouth, like a syrup, using a plastic spoon or syringe (do not use metal).

Dose for option 2:
> » Children between 2 and 5 years: 5 ml of structured silver.
> » People from 6 years and older: 10 ml of structured silver.
> » We can take it hourly if there is a sudden dysentery. It is great for PANDAS/PANS/PITAND cases as well. I have used it hourly with 1oz/30ml 16 times a day.

Structured Silver and Bacteria

The structured silver has a remarkable ability to selectively destroy pathogenic bacteria without causing harm to healthy, friendly flora bacteria. Here I am showing the effectiveness of silver against bacteria, exploring which silver technologies are most effective against bacteria, and providing answers to frequently asked questions about silver and bacteria.

DOES STRUCTURED SILVER REALLY WORK AGAINST BACTERIA?

Study 1: Structured silver on seven pathogens

Recent testing of silver technologies was conducted at Nelson Laboratories, a pharmaceutical-grade laboratory located in Salt Lake City. Nelson Laboratories is FDA registered and third party accredited to ISO 17025 (ACLASS) standards. Nelson Laboratories is a LPG, GMP and GTP facility.

This study provides primary research to answer frequently asked questions from current physicians and the general public. The primary objective of this study was to test the ability of the structured silver to kill pathogens from each of the major categories of pathogenic bacteria along with common yeast. A secondary objective was to test the effectiveness of the 2011 structured alkaline silver technology with the leading silver aquasol technology of the previous decade. This comparative test only included experimentation with two bacterial strains.

The results of this test were clear: structured alkaline silver technology is effective with all major categories of pathogenic bacteria, as well as candida.

Based on the data, the conclusions are the following:

"Structured silver destroys all categories of bacterial and yeast pathogens in 5 minutes and does so at a level of 99.99%, while acidic silver aquasol only destroys 92% in 5 minutes. This means that there were 1,400,000 live MRSA bacteria left in the acidic silver aquasol after five minutes and none in the alkaline structured silver."

Kill Rate (5 Minutes)

Pathogen	Control	Silver Aquasol	Structured Silver
Staphylococcus aureus	0%	92.00%	99.90%
MRSA	0%	92.00%	99.89%
Pseudomonas aeruginosa	0%		99.93%
E-coli	0%		99.91%
Salmonella	0%		99.99%
Candida albicans	0%		99.97%
Streptococcus	0%		99.99%

STUDY 2: SILVER VS. SILVER

A second study comparing silver technologies was conducted at the Brigham Young University laboratory in May 2014. This study compared five silvers of very different concentrations and their ability to kill MRSA, a form of drug-resistant staphylococcus. Two plants had a concentration of 10 ppm, two had 30 ppm and one had 200 ppm. This "apples versus oranges" study showed that only one of the lower concentration silvers kept pace with the structured silver, which was 6 to 20 times more concentrated.

It is important to note that the results of this study were estimated. Quoting the article:

"The counts were so high that the number of CFU had to be estimated at a 1:10,000 dilution of the reaction mixture. Therefore, the log reduction and percentage death values are also estimates."

That being said, here are the test results (MRSA removal rate after 2 minutes):

1. "Solution C" (200 ppm) – 99.999955%
2. "Solution A" (30 ppm) – 99.82%
3. "Solution D" (10-30 ppm) – 58.3%
4. "Solution B" (10-30 ppm) – 47.1%
5. "Solution E" (10-30 ppm) – 39.7%

Thus, two solutions (C and A) killed almost all of the bacteria within two minutes, while three solutions (D, B and E) killed approximately half of the bacteria.

The identity of the solutions of lower concentration is the following:

» Solution A: (Alkaline) Structured silver technology developed in 2011.
» Solutions D, B and E: leading brands of colloidal silver and silver aquasol

It is important to note that the use of 200 ppm silver is generally not recommended, as the volume of silver ingested would quickly exceed the maximum daily silver intake (RfD) recommended by the EPA. Why risk using 200 ppm silver when a much lower concentration structured silver does the same job?

Answers to four common questions

Doctors and the general public frequently ask the following four questions when learning about silver's ability to kill pathogenic bacteria:

1. Why is silver antibacterial?
2. How can silver kill "bad bacteria" but not "good bacteria"?
3. What happens to silver with normal, healthy cells?
4. How can new forms of silver outperform older silvers?

STRUCTURED SILVER/SILVER IS NOT A HEAVY METAL.

Question #1: Why is the silver element antibacterial?

"What happens to the money? I see that silver coins kill bacteria, even in a jar of water. I see that silver in many different forms destroys bad odor, viruses, bacteria... What does silver have and why does it work?

On a chemical diagram, this is what silver looks like. We have two electrons in an inner orbital, 8, 18, and then in the outer orbital we only have one electron. I have indicated it there. This is important and is why silver works. Here it only has one electron, and it spins like an unbalanced wheel. It can never be balanced, even no matter how dense it is, until an electron is placed in this location.

Where are you going to get an electron from? A single electron? It's going to steal it from the bacteria. It will steal it from the viruses. It's going to steal it from the yeast. Yeah! Here is a single-layer cellular organism. I mean, there's just all these tiny little electrons here, and that makes up a cell wall. It is an incomplete cell wall because it is only one electron thick. As soon as this silver particle, which is magnetic, comes close to this bacteria, it will steal it and make the silver completely in balance. Stealing an electron from bacteria, viruses and yeast balances the silver. That's why money works.

There are other mechanisms of action, but silver steals an electron to balance itself, thus destroying pathogens.

The question is: "now that silver has stolen an electron from a bacteria, causing it to die, it is now in equilibrium. What good is it for us medically now?

The point is that once it steals an electron and is balanced, it is ionic silver. That's colloidal silver from the past. Those are the inferior silvers that literally need a silver particle to steal an electron, and now it's neutral and balanced and can't steal any more.

Until it reaches the same proximity with multiple silver molecules. Then, in a crystalline structure, it has the ability to give, take, give, take, and even shoot electrons in a way that kills pathogens.

This is important because we have discovered that this single can become multiple and can come in a tetrahedral circle or in a tetrahedral structure, and we call that crystal structure. So, if we take silver, which is "Ag," and we take four of them, and we put all the oxygens that balance it in here as well, then each one of them has an oxygen and each one has a hydrogen, and suddenly we get a structure crystalline, with hydrogen, oxygen and silver. We call this crystal structure, and this silver particle can easily steal an electron, and then recharge this, and then it can steal an electron, and recharge this, and then it can steal an electron, recharging this. As you can see, a crystalline structure is like a rapid-fire machine gun, killing, killing, killing, killing, while ionic and lower forms of silver only kill one particle for every molecule of silver that exists. That is why the old silver came out of the solution and could cause argyria. New forms of silver don't have the ability to do that because all the silver stays bound to water, how can it get out of solution and cause argyria? Which is the bluish color of the skin."

Question #2: How can silver kill pathogenic bacteria but not healthy bacteria?

"The question is: how can silver destroy bad bacteria while selectively preserving good bacteria?"

In other words, why does it kill pathogens like strep, staphylococcus, pseudomonas, and yeast, but not kill our good gut flora?

Here's why: If this is my silver and it is in a complex or crystal structure, this structured silver is important because it will steal an electron. And we talked about that in a previous video. So, what happens if I steal an electron from this bacteria is that it actually breaks apart and the contents spill out; the bacteria dies. Because this membrane is one electron thick, it's easy to steal an electron, break it like a water balloon, and it just gushes out, the immune system cleaning it all up.

Now, healthy bacteria are different. When we talk about healthy bacteria, we talk about bacterial classifications or nomenclature. What that means is that a bacteria is labeled by a genus, or its genetic makeup, and then by its species. So, we have lactobacillus and then acidophilus, which would be good, healthy bacteria.

The genetic label, lactobacillus, all bacteria labeled lactobacillus, are labeled because they secrete milk fat around themselves to protect themselves. So, from their inner lining, they secrete, like an excretion layer, so what you have is like an "M&M" candy for example, here's the smooth milk chocolate and an extra layer around it to protect it from the acid that's in your stomach. You see, these are healthy, they are found in your intestines, and they need protection from the acids in your stomach. They have learned to do it, evolved, or created it, making this dairy fat surround them.

Silver is soluble in water. Water and fats do not mix. They separate. A bacteria with a single electron shell around it easily loses an electron and dies, but good, healthy bacteria are genetically different with a second shell. And water or silver that comes into contact with it will not penetrate the grease. The fat layer is a barrier for silver to penetrate. It's that easy.

The same can be said for every cell in your body if it is healthy. All our healthy cells are made up of a double lipid layer. Lipid means fat, bilayer means two. So, each cell in your body doesn't just have one layer, it has two and they are made of fats so that water doesn't penetrate.

The simple answer to why silver liquids and gels don't kill good, healthy, friendly bacteria is because they can't penetrate a double layer of fat because they are soluble in water, but they easily steal electrons that are only one electron thick, in bacteria. pathogenic and harmful to health.

Question #3: What happens to silver and healthy cells?

"How does silver, in its liquid, water-soluble form, actually get into a healthy red blood cell or a healthy cell? Because some people are concerned that if it can't get into a fat-covered cell found in the intestines, it may not get into a cell that's in the normal part of healthy tissue, so here's what happens there.

Take a red blood cell as an example. A red blood cell is manufactured by the bone marrow and consists of a double lipid layer. What that means is that you have two layers, and it protects all the contents. Nothing, in the form of water, can enter there. You will be blocked; you will be rejected and you will not be able to enter.

So how does the money come in? Silver is a mineral. Silver is the most active energy mineral, meaning it transfers more electricity than any other metal.

Now, what is the manufactured element, the mineral element, of a red blood cell? Iron. You may have heard it said: ferritin, which is ferrous or ferrous oxide. All these words mean that this cell is made of iron. So, if you have iron, which makes up a quarter of that entire cell, it will disperse throughout this cell and in the hemoglobin, which means iron, there will be iron. Iron has a specific charge that attracts silver.

Maybe you've seen this in your home wiring, where you have a wire, that's copper, right next to it, after the insulation, there's a silver wire. Because? These are the two best conductors of electricity, and since your body is an electromagnet, these copper particles attract the silver particles, so when the silver comes and hits them, it now wants to be attracted to that cell, but, even so, it doesn't. Isn't it until it is actively transported, and what is actively transported across the membrane of a red blood cell?

You have enzymes. Various enzymes that basically open the pores and allow the silver to come in because it helps balance or complete this electromagnet called hemoglobin.

Silver is actively transported to iron and binds to iron inside the cell, and that is why silver, in its small particle form, can get into a red blood cell and not into healthy bacteria, because the healthy bacteria They do not have iron or any other metal that absorbs them.

In fact, if you take copper and put it in the same area as silver and put it in an acid, that's what a battery does. Two separate metals, in an acid, form a battery. This is how the energy of your cells increases with silver. Now, those of you who are doctors and want to try this on yourself, it's very simple. If you swallow silver and take four times the normal dose, if it destroys your good, healthy lactobacillus or your good flora in your intestines, you would know because it would cause diarrhea. The evidence is that when you take tetracycline or when you take other antibiotics, it kills the good bacteria and produces, in about 12 to 24 hours, diarrhea. So, if you want to take a quadruple dose of silver, swallow it and when you don't have diarrhea, you'll know these are facts, not just theories."

Question #4: Do all silvers work the same: ionic, colloidal, hydrosol and structured silver?

"The question is: why is silver in structured form more valuable than silver in ionic or colloidal form?"

It's that simple: if you took silver and a silver atom, and let's call it right here. That's money.

Now, let's say that can steal an electron from this bacteria. That's great, that dies, but now it's neutral, unless we add enough energy to this simple silver particle that it now becomes energetic enough that there are four silver particles attached together and they bring with them a complete structure of oxygen and hydrogen. Because two hydrogens and one oxygen are water, you're now structuring the silver in a situation where you have hydrogen and oxygen, and by doing that in each of them, you end up with a structure where they share electrons.

Then they join together and, as silver normally lacks an electron, now, when they join together, they share it. And they share with oxygen, so it becomes a crystalline structure. And in certain scientific articles by Rustum Roy, he mentions that Ag, or silver, 4O4, which is this right here, is a very valuable pathogen killer. But, because it's in water, and there's all this hydrogen and oxygen everywhere, and other silver particles, it only exists for about a second, maybe, and then it turns into Ag6, or Ag5, or Ag12, or Ag1, because there is so much water, it separates it, it joins it again, it separates it, it joins it again.

But when we add enough energy, right here, for it to become structured water, a matrix forms that holds it in place longer, so 40% of the time, we have these crystalline structured silvers ready to kill unlike other hydrosols that only kill for a ten-thousandth of a second and then leave the solution and re-enter.

Now, unlike single silver which only kills one bacteria at a time, it becomes totally neutral after a death, so, I've said this before, ionic, colloidal and other silver are basically a one-shot revolver. Shooting. A shot, a death, are neutral. But when you put it in a structure that includes oxygens and hydrogens, now you have the ability to steal an electron, right here, and send it a charge, which can then steal an electron, send a charge, send a charge, all of these have charges.

Where does the extra electron end up going? In fact, it ends up getting into the oxygen, and the oxygen is already saturated, and it fires like a rapid-fire machine gun, one silver electron at a time, and steals one too. So now this crystal structure is stealing an electron and, one ten-thousandth of a second later, it's throwing one toward a bacteria. Steal, shoot, steal, shoot, make this structure more and more energetic, exposing oxygen, which kills pathogens like cancer cells, like virus cells, like bacteria cells.

These unique oxygens are released all the time, and you get multiple methods of killing with structured silver. And put it in an alkaline system that your body recognizes and can use every day.

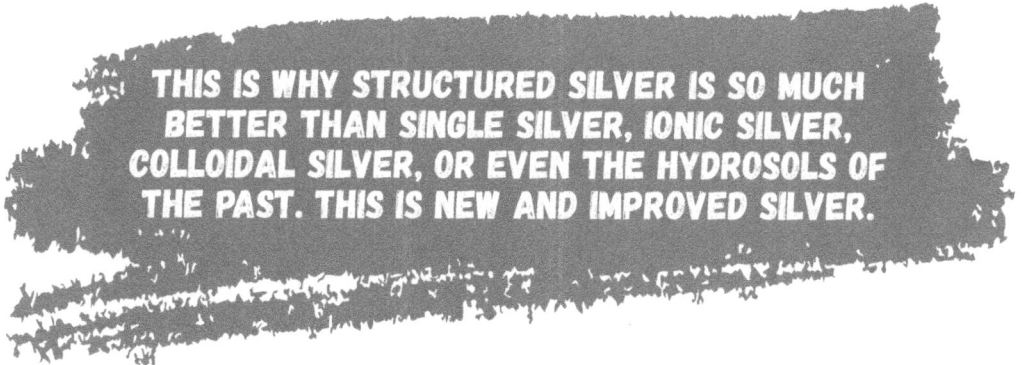

THIS IS WHY STRUCTURED SILVER IS SO MUCH BETTER THAN SINGLE SILVER, IONIC SILVER, COLLOIDAL SILVER, OR EVEN THE HYDROSOLS OF THE PAST. THIS IS NEW AND IMPROVED SILVER.

Structured silver vs. Colloidal silver

Historically, silver has been used to purify water. Today, international airliners and NASA use silver to purify water. At the end of the 19th century, the uses of silver in medicine began to be documented in scientific journals. The purifying properties of silver are well established. The main question is: what is the best delivery system?

The body functions best in an alkaline state. Many studies show that bad bacteria and yeast cannot thrive when the body is alkaline, compared to an acidic state. Unfortunately, most colloidal silvers are acidic and not alkaline. In addition to acidity, one of the other main concerns with colloidal silver is that the elemental silver will break away from the suspension and build up in the bottle. If this happens in the bottle, it can also happen in the body and build up.

The solution is to use silver bound to structured water at a specific energy frequency instead of a colloidal suspension. When silver is added to structured water, it becomes part of the water molecule rather than simply being suspended in the water. The structured silver solution is not acidic but is balanced at an alkaline pH of 7.4. It will not be metabolized or accumulate in the body because silver is part of the water molecule.

Water is what the human body depends on for all its functions and, ultimately, its survival. Researchers are finding that structured water is better absorbed by the body's cells than purified or distilled water. Structured water also creates a positive aerobic environment through stable, free oxygen. This promotes healthy bacteria and nullifies bad bacteria that thrive in an anaerobic state. Water in nature is also naturally structured. The potential benefits of structured water are improved metabolism, strengthened DNA, more energy, and a better ability to hydrate cells. When silver is combined with structured water, it becomes a powerful one-two punch.

Silver is not a toxic, heavy metal like lead, mercury, arsenic, and cadmium. Gold is heavy based on density, yet it is not a toxic metal.

Digestive Enzymes

Betaine HCl

» Is an acidic version of betaine that works as hydrochloric acid (HCl) in your stomach.
» HCl breaks down food
» Low HCl in the stomach means high levels of gut infections like SIBO.
» Low HCl results in impaired nutrient absorption thus leading to low calcium, magnesium, iron, and B12, which leads to conditions like anemia which are common in autism and most autoimmune diseases.
» Low HCl means we will have impaired digestive function in the esophagus and small intestine.

Adequate levels of HCl kill bacteria before they enter the small intestine.

When HCl is low there will be constipation/bloating and belching.

People with low HCl or people with autoimmune conditions like H. Pylori infections, and anemia, over those over 65 years of age people who use antacids or proton pump inhibitors.

Symptoms of low stomach acid (HCl) are burping, bloating, sensation of excessive fullness, reflux, heartburn, and indigestion.

- » HCl is known to be helpful in healing ulcers.
- » Low betaine and homocysteine levels can cause heart attack and stroke.
- » Betaine improves muscle mass, growth, strength, and tone. It also increases stamina.
- » Betaine helps to metabolize proteins.

Betaine shows the ability to break down and remove fats. Thus, helping the liver to detoxify by protecting the body from the damage of toxin exposure helping the liver to remove the toxins and chemicals.

Betaine protects the liver against hepatotoxic effects from medications, pesticides, and herbicides.

Betaine reduces muscle aches and pains as well as joint tissue damage.

Betaine is an important amino acid for the prevention of chronic diseases. It also protects the internal organs and enhances their performance.

- » It helps treat depression.
- » Powerful digestive acid.
- » High HCl helps nutrients to be absorbed.
- » Low HCl causes lack of nutrition and causes gastritis, asthma, candida, Rheumatic arthritis, and arteriosclerosis.
- » People with low HCl in the body are prone to parasitic and bacterial infections. People with acne, yeast infections, gallstones, and allergies do not produce enough HCl.

Supplementing with betaine HCl can help with the following:

- » Anemia
- » Arteriosclerosis
- » Acne
- » Diarrhea
- » Stomach ulcers
- » Inner ear infections
- » Yeast infections

- » Malabsorption of nutrients
- » Gastroesophageal reflux disease
- » Indigestion and heartburn
- » Stomach disorders
- » Food sensitivities/allergies
- » Thyroid issues
- » Gallstones

Oxbile

Helps to digest fats and promote the absorption of fat-soluble vitamins. Prevents gallstones, SIBO, and harmful dysbiosis

- » Reduces constipation
- » Decreases inflammation

Symptoms of deficiency in bile:

- » Sluggish digestion
- » Heavy feeling after a meal
- » Stomach pain and bloating
- » Fat-soluble vitamin deficiency
- » Constipation
- » Pale or fatty stools
- » Jaundice
- » Gallstones
- » Poor detoxification
- » Dry skin or psoriasis

Pancriatin

- » Digest fats, proteins, and sugars
- » Helps with loose, fatty stools.
- » Hekos with the absorption of vitamins and minerals
- » Promotes healthy weight.

Bromelain

For digestive disorders, allergies, and recovery from injury.

Protease Enzyme

For the digestion of proteins for the absorption of amino acids.

Papain

Enzyme extracted from the raw fruit of the papain plant. Breaks down proteins, peptides, and amino acids.

» Reduces inflammation and pain
» Aids in digestion
» Fights infections
» Anti-tumor effect
» Wound healing
» Supports a healthy immune system
» Supports a healthy inflammatory response

In 2016 an amazing man and dear friend, Dr Roby Mitchell, RIP opened my eyes by introducing me to the book by Dr Jonathan Wright named "Why Stomach Acid Is Good for You."

What are the symptoms of low stomach acid (HCl). Low stomach acid is called hypochloridria.

» Low amino acid
» Low minerals
» Low B vitamins
» Heartburn
» GERD
» Depression
» Anxiety
» Insomnia
» Fungal overgrowth

Bacteria die in the acid bath of the stomach. Bacteria overgrowth in the stomach and small intestine leads to symptoms such as gas, constipation, diarrhea, and increased susceptibility to potentially fatal infections like cholera and salmonella.

» Poor absorption of vitamins, minerals, and a/c.
» Poor digestion of proteins
» Allergies
» Asthma
» Pernicious anemia
» Stomach cancer
» Skin issues like acne, dermatitis, eczema, and urticaria (hives)
» Gallstones
» Rheumatoid arthritis
» Lupus
» Graves disease
» Ulcerative colitis
» Hepatitis
» Osteoporosis
» Type 1 diabetes (insulin-dependent)
» Accelerated aging

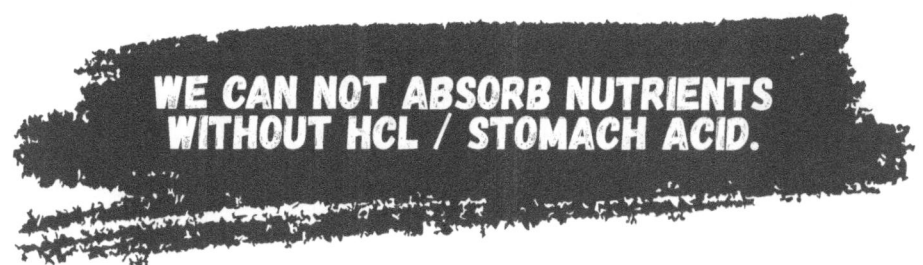

WE CAN NOT ABSORB NUTRIENTS WITHOUT HCL / STOMACH ACID.

SUPPLEMENTATION ROUTINE

NAME: **ATEC:**   **DATE:**

SCHEDULE	SUPPLEMENT	DOSAGE	TIME	COMMENTS
UPON AWAKENING				
BREAKFAST				
MID MORNING				
LUNCH				
MID AFTERNOON				
DINNER				
BEDTIME				

NOTES:

CELEBRATE YOUR CHILD'S SMALL VICTORIES, THEY ARE
JUST AS IMPORTANT AS THE BIG ONES.

Chapter 6
Parasite
Protocol (PP)

- Recommendations
- Parasite Protocol (PP)
- Dosage tables
- Frequent questions

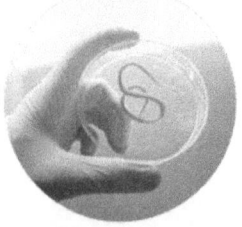

Parasite Protocol (PP)

» In order to stop the reproductive cycle of the parasites, it is suggested to carry out the PP until the ATEC reaches 0. Each cycle consists of 21 days and begins two days before the full moon each month.

» It is suggested that PP be done by all family members and pets to avoid reinfection. The family can do short rounds of 5 or 7 days. Pets should be treated by a veterinarian.

» Please review the dosage charts below.

» Mebendazole should be purchased in "Tablets/Pills" presentation, avoid buying the liquid presentation, as they contain dyes, flavoring, and sugar.

» If you are taking: Tagamet, Ethotoin, Penicillin, Zithromax, Amoxicillin, Mephenytoin (Mesantoin), Carbamazepine, Flagyl (Metronidazole) you should consult with your doctor if you can do deworming with MEBENDAZOLE, since there is interaction between them, especially with Flagyl (Metronidazole) and Tagamet (Cimetidine). It is my opinion that flagyl should not be used by anyone with autism. Antibiotics in general set back the recovery by months. It is like throwing a wrench into a running motor.

» The enema plays a fundamental role in this treatment, since it allows the elimination of toxins released by the parasites when they die. In addition, it prevents the reabsorption of toxins in the body. Enemas also help to remove the dead parasites that are sticking to the intestines. A dead parasite in the intestine can be more toxic than when it is alive. We begin absorbing the toxins from the parasites. Parasites carry other pathogens on them like candida, virus, bacteria as well as toxic heavy metals. For this reason, enemas are a crucial part of the process during the PP.

Parasite Protocol (PP)

Mebendazole:

Take (1) one dose two (2) times a day, with food (breakfast and dinner), from day 1 to day 21. It can be given at the same time as the Humic/Fulvic, black seed oil, and the "chondroitin sulfate/oleic acid/D" during meals.

EACH CYCLE CONSISTS OF 21 DAYS AND BEGINS TWO DAYS BEFORE THE FULL MOON EACH MONTH.

Stone Breaker:

Take (1) one dose twice daily with food, from day 1 to day 21. This can be given with mebendazole and the other supplements at the same time.

Castor oil:

Take one (1) dose every other day during breakfast with other supplements or when your child returns from school if they go to school. Normally, it goes with breakfast. And only give what they tolerate. Castor oil may cause diarrhea at higher than tolerated doses. People with constipation may benefit from higher doses of the castor oil.

Enemas:

The frequency of the enemas will depend on each case. If your child is uncomfortable, upset, anxious, or anything out of the ordinary in the morning or afternoon, you can do the enema at that time. Otherwise, it is best to do the enemas between 4 and 7 pm. That way you are home for the remainder of the day. If there is any water up higher in the intestine and comes out later than the first release, then we don't have an uncomfortable situation in the car or in a store.

Mebendazole Implants (optional):

These implants are a quick measure to relieve anal itching caused by pinworms which are small, threadlike white worms that can live in the large intestine and rectum. During sleep, the females of these worms emerge from the rectum and lay their eggs on the skin around the anus, causing intense itching. They can also be used in cases of high parasite load. You can put a diaper cream on the area in order to calm the itching until the parasitic infection has cleared up with the PP.

To use Mebendazole implants, crush one Mebendazole tablet completely (100mg tablet) and dilute it in 10 to 30 ml of water. Then, draw up the mixture into a small 10-30ml syringe (without needle). While the child is sleeping, insert only the tip of the syringe into the anus and inject the liquid into the colon, remove the syringe, and allow the introduced liquid to take effect overnight while your child sleeps. The next morning, do an enema to ensure that the toxins and waste released by the now dead parasites are removed. Repeat this procedure every night until the anal itching disappears and the parasite load decreases. The implant can be done with a syringe (no needle) or a pear.

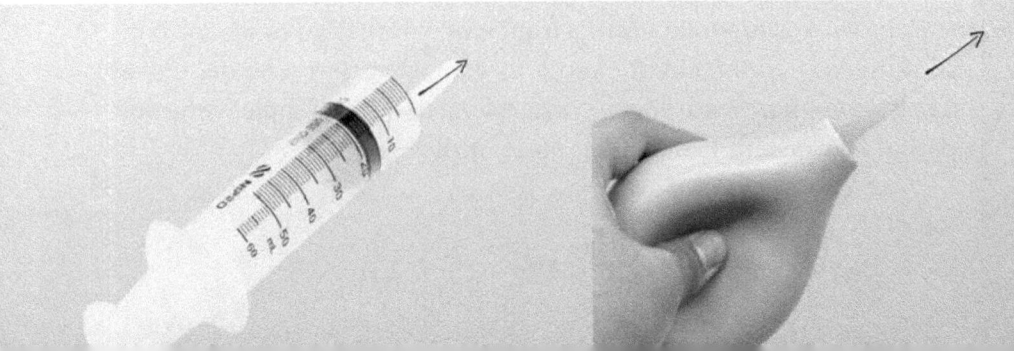

Mebendazol: (1) one dose two (2) times a day, with meals (breakfast and dinner).

Weight in kg	Weight in lb	Dose	Indications
11	25	25 mg	2 x day
23	50	50 mg	2 x day
35	70	100 mg	2 x day
43+	100+	200 mg	2 x day

Stone Breaker: (1) one dose two (2) times a day, with meals (breakfast and dinner).

Weight in kg	Weight in lb	Dose	Indications
11	25	5 drops	2 x day
23	50	12 drops	2 x day
35	70	15 drops	2 x day
42	100+	22 drops	2 x day

DOSAGE IN POUNDS AND KILOGRAMS

ALL DOSAGE TABLES ARE EXPRESSED IN BOTH POUNDS AND KILOGRAMS TO MEET THE PREFERENCES OF FAMILIES AROUND THE WORLD. CHOOSE THE OPTION THAT IS MOST SUITABLE FOR YOUR COUNTRY. IF THERE IS A CONFUSION, EMAIL ME AT KERRI@KERRIRIVERA.COM

Castor Oil

The main objective of the use of castor oil in the Parasite Protocol (PP) is to remove the parasite, liver fluke, a parasite that lodges itself in the liver. We do not use it with the intention of it being a laxative, although it is important to mention that it can have laxative effects, which can be beneficial in cases of constipation.

Importantly, the dosage of castor oil is determined based on individual tolerance and is not related to weight or age. It is recommended to start with a dose between 1/8th and ¼ teaspoon and gradually increase every two days until you find the dose that generates a smooth bowel movement, avoiding diarrhea. There are people with constipation who tolerate up to 2 spoons a day. There are others who tolerate only 1/8th teaspoon before having diarrhea. Start low and go up slow to find the perfect dose of castor oil.

Frequently asked questions
Parasite Protocol

How long should my child be dewormed?

Once we get into the deworming process, **we must keep in mind the importance of maintaining this cleaning practice throughout our lives to enjoy good and balanced health.** Once the reproductive cycle of the parasites has been interrupted (which can vary from person to person), extensive 21-day deworming cycles will no longer be necessary. You can then perform maintenance cycles every 2 or 3 months, with shorter periods of between 3 to 7 days. However, until the ATEC reaches 0, parasites must be treated in addition to the rest of the CD protocol.

My son won't stop eating, what can I do?

When there is an overpopulation of candida and parasites, very strong levels of anxiety usually occur. They are generally thin but hungry children, wanting to eat large amounts of food all day and almost always looking for high carb foods. The parasites are consuming the sugars which are carbohydrates. Thus, once the parasites and candida are under attack. They look for their sources to survive. That being carbohydrates which are sugars.

To address this situation, the following strategies can be implemented:

> » **Increase CD dose:** Some children may have difficulty tolerating higher doses of CD. In these cases, we give more of the structured silver, which also helps reduce the toxic load of pathogens.

> » **Increase your intake of healthy fats:** Adding a tablespoon of C8/MCT (medium chain triglycerides), beef tallow, lard, duck fat, or casein-free ghee (clarified butter) to each meal is beneficial. Increasing fat helps lower the desire for carbohydrates. As well as feeding the person and not their pathogens.

> » **Increase protein consumption** of animal origin and reduce carbohydrate intake. Helps us to feel full. Once we're full, we don't run around the kitchen looking for more food and carbs.

Inappropriate Behaviors:

Occasionally a child might begin to exhibit behaviors that they did not have before starting protocol or they feel that the behaviors are getting worse. Parasites have a clear goal; they want to survive and reproduce.

They seek to keep their eggs in the host to complete their life cycle. In some cases, behaviors such as playing with feces, nail biting, scratching the anus, putting fingers in one's own or other people's mouths, and/ or spitting might be observed. All of these behaviors are caused by parasites. As we progress in the PP, these behaviors begin to decrease and finally disappear.

To mitigate or counteract these symptoms, it is suggested to administer a double dose of CD while the child is awake. If crying symptoms persist or if the child touches or hits his head a lot, he may have a headache. It is important to remember that most children with autism have difficulties communicating and express their discomfort through behaviors. If the above recommendations are exhausted and the problem persists, the administration of a dose of ibuprofen (not acetaminophen/paracetamol) can be considered.

My son wet the bed, he peed, he didn't do this before... What should I do?

Parasites are living beings and when they feel they are being attacked they become alert because they know that their life is in danger, so they attack to show their dissatisfaction by releasing toxins, including a substance similar to morphine, which makes their children not feel like they need to urinate. or that they are urinating. This is not the child's fault; it is just part of the parasite elimination process. It is a temporary symptom.

Chapter 7
Chelation of heavy metals

- Zeolite
- Bentonite Baths
- EDTA
- Humic/Fulvic
- PektiClean

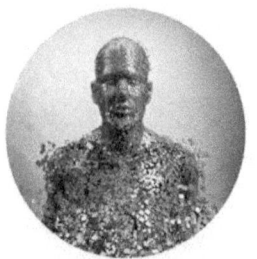

Chelation of heavy metals

Heavy metal chelation is a process where substances called chelators are used to eliminate or reduce the presence of heavy metals in the body. Heavy metals, such as lead, mercury, cadmium or aluminum, are toxic and cause damage to the body and brain.

Chelators are compounds that have the ability to bind heavy metals and form stable compounds that can be easily eliminated from the body through urine, feces, sweat and hair. By grabbing onto heavy metals, chelators prevent them from accumulating in different organs and tissues, which helps prevent or reduce harmful health effects.

Heavy metal chelation is used as a treatment for heavy metal poisoning or to reduce the toxic metal load in people exposed to high levels of these compounds. It is also used in detoxification therapies and as a preventive measure in certain cases. There are heavy metals in the biofilms that exist in the intestine and in the blood. Children with autism have biofilms, so they all have heavy metals, and we have to use chelators as part of the complete healing protocol.

The Chelators used in the CD Protocol

ZEOLITE

Zeolite, particularly clinoptilolite, is a rare natural mineral formed by the chemical reaction between volcanic ash and seawater. The benefits of zeolite are due to its crystalline structure; Zeolites are porous and negatively charged, allowing for the selective removal of toxins, especially heavy metals, which are positively charged. Simply put, a zeolite detox involves this mineral acting as a detoxification filter by grabbing toxic heavy metals, trapping them within its structure and passing them through the body via the excretory system.

How does zeolite detoxify the body?

Numerous scientific studies attest to the selective nature of clinoptilolite zeolite's ability to eliminate toxins. By taking a liquid zeolite supplement sized for absorption through the digestive tract, this beneficial mineral absorbs toxins from the body. Imagine zeolite as a negatively charged magnet, most harmful toxins are positively charged and opposites attract. Zeolite attracts and traps positively charged toxins such as lead, mercury, arsenic, cadmium and many more, and removes them from the body through the excretory system.

Zeolite crystal structure

A key factor in zeolite's effectiveness is the mineral's crystal structure. The mineral itself is a network of tetrahedra linked by oxygen atoms that form a network-like structure. Imagine a honeycomb, but on a microscopic scale. This network-like structure of each zeolite particle is made up of uniformly shaped pores or channels into which substances can be absorbed. As liquid passes through these pores, the channels act as sieves or filters for the molecules, allowing the zeolites to "capture" positively charged toxins in what is known as cation exchange.

The unique structure and charge of clinoptilolite zeolite provides detoxification in two ways. The first, as mentioned above, is the absorption or capture of toxins within the zeolite. The second method is through adsorption, where the toxins adhere to the outside of the zeolite particle. In this way, zeolite acts as one of the most effective natural detoxifiers on the planet.

The benefits of zeolite detox

There are many types of zeolites found in nature, but the clinoptilolite zeolite is the most suitable for therapeutic applications. Through scientific research, zeolite has been evaluated for removal of environmental toxins, shown to promote health and well-being in numerous animal studies, and demonstrated benefits for detoxification, immune health, antioxidant support, and intestinal health in humans.

The remarkable detoxifying effects of clinoptilolite zeolite were observed in research conducted with rodents. In this trial, lead-poisoned mice were treated with clinoptilolite zeolite and showed an 89% reduction in % in lead accumulation in the liver, a reduction of 91 % lead in the kidneys and a reduction of 77 % lead in bones.

Given the known harmful health effects of lead, including its impact on brain development in children, clinoptilolite zeolite may be a natural and safe way to help detoxify lead and other heavy metals from the body.

A wide range of clinical and preclinical trials in live subjects, as well as in vitro or Petri dish laboratory settings, show promise for the many benefits of zeolite. Recent research points to many potential beneficial applications of clinoptilolite zeolite, particularly its ability to absorb heavy metals, provide immune support by scavenging free radicals, and support the gut microbiome.

Zeolite Clinoptilolite and Heavy Metals

Clinoptilolite zeolite is widely recognized as a heavy metal detoxifier. Today, many people turn to micronized zeolite to help remove harmful and toxic substances from the gastrointestinal tract, including heavy metals, as well as nitrosamines, ammonia, mycotoxins, radioactive materials, and pesticides.

In a clinical investigation using rats as subjects, researchers found that the natural zeolite clinoptilolite effectively removed aluminum from the plasma, liver, and bones of rats intoxicated with aluminum chloride.

A clinical study evaluated human subjects and found statistically significant improvements in blood arsenic levels after twelve weeks of zeolite treatment.

Another clinical study evaluating the ability of micronized clinoptilolite zeolite (small particles) to remove heavy metals from humans demonstrated that zeolite increased excretion of heavy metals through urine without loss of beneficial electrolyte minerals.

Immune Support and Gut Health

The body's immune system is influenced by both external and internal systems. When it comes to the gut's role in immune function, zeolite has been shown to help improve the integrity of the intestinal barrier, causing a positive impact on the intestinal ecosystem, thereby supporting the immune system.

In a randomized, double-blind, placebo-controlled trial, 52 resistance-trained men and women, ages 20 to 50, received a zeolite regimen for 12 weeks. The conclusion showed beneficial effects on the integrity of the intestinal wall indicated by reduced concentrations of zonulin, a protein that increases the permeability of the tight junctions between cells in the wall of the digestive tract, also known as "leaky gut."

In terms of our overall well-being and quality of life, researchers have hypothesized that due to zeolite's positive impacts on the gut microbiome, it indirectly benefits the gut-brain connection at the central nervous system level. For example, in one study, the zeolite clinoptilolite was shown to reduce stress and improve sleep, although more research is needed to better understand the connection between zeolite supplementation and overall mood in humans.

By helping the body eliminate heavy metals and promoting balance in the intestine, clinoptilolite zeolite promotes overall homeostasis. Overall, research shows that clinoptilolite zeolite is a highly effective detoxifier, supports the immune system, demonstrates antioxidant effects, and promotes overall well-being.

Liquid zeolite or powder zeolite

The various zeolite supplements available today include liquid and powder supplements. Although it may seem that everything simply boils down to preferences, in reality there are substantial differences between the two. Firstly, zeolite powder is usually a crude substance that contains toxins found naturally in the environment during mining. It is necessary for the zeolite to go through a liquid purification process to eliminate toxins and be able to be effectively detoxified once ingested.

Secondly, purified liquid zeolite can be reduced to nanometer particle size so that it can be absorbed at the cellular level, since non-micronized zeolite cannot be absorbed through water or fats. These nanosized particles are stored in liquid suspension as this is the preferred medium for the zeolite and ensures that the zeolite can travel throughout the body to completely detoxify it.

Lastly, most zeolites are not lab tested, preventing the consumer from truly understanding what is in their products. Laboratory testing is the best way to know that the product is free of existing toxins so that it can work as a detoxifier in the body.

There are 15 key reasons why DHQ Enhanced Purified Activated Liquid Zeolite is the most unique and extraordinary dietary supplement on the market today!

1. Extremely safe and non-toxic: Purified activated liquid zeolite is not toxic at all and is removed safely and completely after 5 to 7 hours. The toxins it captures in its cage are effectively deactivated so that there are no side effects as they are eliminated from the body; It is important to drink plenty of water (8 to 10 glasses a day) when taking zeolite. And because most medications are negatively charged chemicals, purified activated liquid zeolite tends to leave them alone.

2. Removes Toxic Heavy Metals: Purified liquid activated zeolite has the perfect molecular structure to adhere to and then remove heavy metals (including radioactive ones) from the body, including mercury, cadmium, lead, arsenic, aluminum, strontium and excess iron.

3. Helps eliminate pesticides, herbicides and dioxins: these chemicals are the main candidates for causing cancer and altering hormonal balance; It is very important that they are eliminated from the body as quickly as possible.

4. Reduces viral load: Purified activated liquid zeolite adheres to viral components. This can help relieve some of the symptoms of viral illnesses and infections.

5. Reduces the absorption of nitrosamines: These substances can be found in processed meats, bacon, sausages, cold cuts, etc. and are related to pancreatic, stomach and colon cancer, as well as type II diabetes. Purified liquid activated zeolite helps neutralize these toxins in the digestive tract by capturing them in their molecular cages before they can be absorbed by the body. They are then safely eliminated from the body.

6. Helps buffer the body's pH to achieve healthy alkalinity: Purified liquid activated zeolite acts as a pH buffer, helping to prevent acidic conditions in our blood and cellular fluids that encourage low immunity and disease. An alkaline body creates an inhospitable environment for pathogens. Normalizing the pH in it creates an environment that kills bacteria and viruses.

7. Helps buffer blood sugar: It can also buffer excess glucose due to its negative charge and therefore helps reduce blood sugar spikes.

8. Helps reduce the risk of cancer: Purified liquid activated zeolite eliminates toxins that can cause cancer (75% or more of cancers can be related to toxins).

9. Improves nutrient absorption: Purified liquid activated zeolite also helps reduce incidents of diarrhea, which is why zeolites can now be found in the latest diarrhea medications.

10. Acts as a powerful antioxidant: The cage-like structure of purified activated liquid zeolite can also trap free radical molecules, making it an effective antioxidant.

11. Reduces Allergy Symptoms: Purified liquid activated zeolite can capture some of the antigens that cause allergies, migraines, and asthma and in doing so, helps reduce symptoms.

12. Immune Modulator – May act as an effective "natural" immune modulator. It could effectively regulate an underactive or overactive immune system back to normal. Most illnesses and diseases occur when the immune system is out of balance!

13. Helps prevent premature aging: By eliminating the toxic load with Purified Liquid Activated Zeolite, our body's normal repair and regeneration mechanisms are freed to work efficiently.

14. Extremely easy and pleasant to take: NO MESSY POWDER! Most serious detox solutions are difficult to take, taste unpleasant, and can leave a person feeling exhausted because they also indiscriminately remove healthy minerals. Purified Liquid Activated Zeolite is a small bottle of tasteless liquid that can be taken with or without food and removes only harmful ions.

15. It contains dihydroquercetin (DHQ), also known as taxifolin, which is a bioflavonoid similar in structure to quercetin. Nearly 600 studies conducted over the past 50 years have investigated its effectiveness and safety. Flavonoids perform two important functions...they strengthen the body's immune response and act as powerful super-antioxidants. Flavonoids have been reported to have antiviral, antiallergic, antiplatelet, anti-inflammatory, anti-tumor, and antioxidant activities.

Lead replaces calcium in bones. Lead replaces calcium in the blood, thereby damaging the blood. Lead causes elevated levels of uric acid. It impairs kidney function and causes gout.

Mercury is the most toxic element known to man and is stored in the brain, kidneys and liver.

Cadmium is associated with cancer. Cadmium irritates adrenal activity. 1 of the most toxic metals that affects the kidneys and cardiovascular system.

Arsenic is very toxic. Arsenic affects the left side of the body and the brain. It is high in rice, beer, wine, and butter. Arsenic is found in pesticides used on grapes and fruits. It is an adrenal disruptor.

Why liquid instead of powder/capsules?

Zeolite powder (in capsules) only acts in the intestine. We cannot remove heavy metals from bones, organs, blood and brain with zeolite powder or capsules. Our clean micronized liquid zeolite is ½ micron in size, making it the smallest and most advanced liquid on the market. And all liquid zeolites are smaller than all powders/capsules. This liquid zeolite is transported along 60,000 miles of blood vessels in the circulatory system. Starts working in seconds throughout the body.

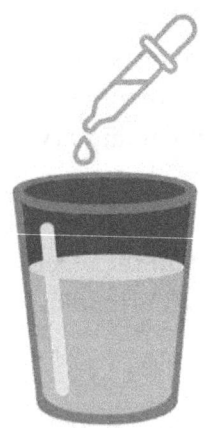

Indications for Ultra Liquid Zeolite:

For cases with normal evacuations or with a tendency to constipation.

Distribute the zeolite drops by weight into 1 to 2 ounces of water. Consume the zeolite three times a day away from food and other supplements. For example, if you need 3 drops, take it 3 times a day, for a total of 9 drops daily.

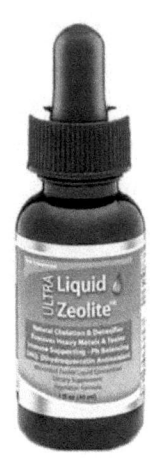

In pounds	In kg	Dose
Up to 25 lb	Up to 11 kg	3 drops - 3 x day
26 lb – 50 lb	12 kg–22 kg	3 drops - 3 x day
51 lb – 75 lb	23 kg – 34 kg	3 drops - 3 x day
76 lb – 100 lb and up	35 kg – 45 kg and up	3 drops - 3 x day

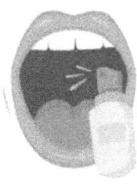

PBX Zeolite spray

Apply the PBX spray directly into the mouth.

In pounds	In kg	Dose
Less than 30 lb	Less than 13.5 kg	1 spray - 3 x day
31 a 69 lb	14 kg – 30kg	2 sprays - 3 x day
70 lb and up	31 kg and up	3 sprays - 3 x day

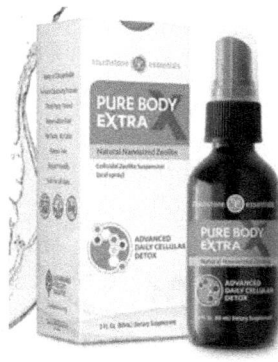

The best zeolite in the market is https://kerririvera.thegoodinside.com/pbpbx-trial-offer/ so good that with this link you pay a special price just to try it. This is the company you trust that you will have important results.

BENTONITE BATHS

Clay baths help eliminate heavy metals through the skin. According to studies, bentonite clay is believed to act through a process called absorption.

Absorption is a phenomenon in which molecules or ions of one substance adhere to the surface of another substance. In the case of bentonite clay, its crystalline structure and high negative charge allow it to act as a molecular sponge. When clay is mixed with water and applied to the skin, its particles attract and adhere to heavy metals present on the skin's surface.

DIRECTIONS FOR MAKING A BENTONITE CLAY BATH:

» Add the bentonite clay to a tub full of water or to a large, plastic tub. Make sure to dissolve it evenly.

» The water should be warm to hot. As in a comfortable temperature for the person.

» Put the child in the tub and make sure the water covers the body from the neck down or as much as possible. It is good to stay in the tub soaking for 10 minutes. Any more than 10 minutes you can risk reabsorption of the metals that the bentonite clay pulled out.

» Then shower as usual to remove any remaining bentonite from your skin. It can cause the skin to become dry. If you see that the skin gets dry. You can always hydrate the skin with black seed oil. Black seed oil is soothing to dry, chapped or burned skin. After towel drying your child. You can moisten your hands with the black seed oil then massage it on the child's skin.

» If the child likes to bathe for a long time, that is fine. During hte last 10 minutes of the bath you can add the bentonite clay.

SUGGESTED USAGE OF
BENTONITE CLAY BY WEIGHT

In pounds	In kg	Dose
25 lb	11 kg	¼ cup
50 lb	22 kg	½ cup
75 lb	34 kg	¾ cup
100 and up	45 kg and up	1 cup

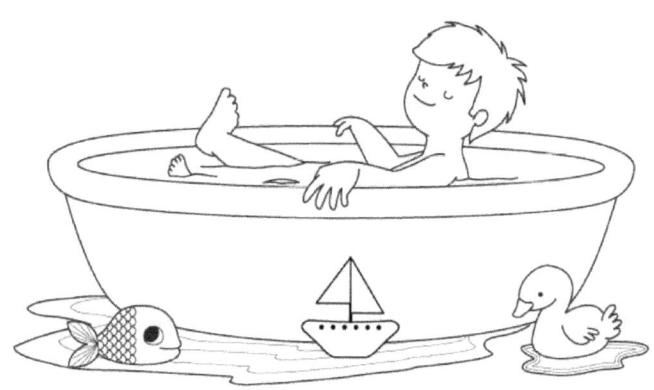

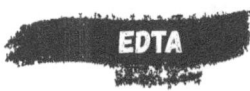

EDTA

It is a versatile chelating agent that forms bonds with metal ions, mostly heavy metals. It is very safe so it can be taken by anyone for long or indefinite periods of time. It has no side effects.

It is a support supplement for ASD, Alzheimer's, heart disease or anyone living in today's toxic world.

EDTA oral chelation should be started with minimal doses and increase gradually. Due to the fact that this supplement eliminates heavy metals in a general way. Wherever heavy metals are present, there is also candida. When the chelator removes the toxic heavy metals, it can leave some free candida. We want to make sure that we have our other supplements in already for candida like CD, BSO (black seed oil), SSS (structured silver solution), Humic/fulvic and berberine. They all help us to control the pathogen load in the body.

For this reason, the suggested starting time for heavy metal chelation is after the third parasite protocol has been completed. This is to ensure that the toxic load has been considerably reduced and that we do not have to suffer Herxheimer symptoms. Start with a low dose and depending on your child's tolerance and reaction, gradually increase the dose until you reach the suggested dose based on your child's weight.

Suggested use:

Dilute EDTA drops in water (1oz/30ml or 2oz/60ml of water) separate from food at least 10 to 15 minutes prior. But if you can be close to a CD dose, separate only 10 minutes from a CD dose. Example: If you give CD at 2:00 pm you can give EDTA or zeolite at 2:10 pm. CD neutralizes heavy metals. So, giving a chelator after a dose of cd is a great idea.

In pounds	In kg	Dose
25 lb	11 kg	6 drops 3 x day
50 lb	22 kg	12 drops 3 x day
75 lb	34 kg	18 drops 3 x day
100 and up	45 kg and up	24 drops 3 day

HUMIC/FULVIC

Humic/Fulvic is a combination of humic and fulvic acids, organic nutrients extracted from virgin and ancient soils. These compounds contain a diversity of essential nutrients, including amino acids, minerals, nucleic acids, and phytochemical compounds. It has been used in Ayurvedic medicine and has been shown to have beneficial health properties by improving nutrient absorption, balancing the gut microbiome, supporting the immune system, and facilitating the elimination of toxins from the body. It crosses the blood-brain barrier and removes heavy metals from the brain, among other benefits.

Benefits of Humic/Fulvic:

» Improves nutrient absorption at the cellular level.
» Balances the intestinal microbiome.
» Increases blood oxygenation.
» Support the immune system.
» Reduces inflammation.
» Facilitates the elimination of toxins from the body.
» Crosses the blood-brain barrier and removes heavy metals from the brain.
» Seals leaky gut.
» Regulates the bioavailability of iron, calcium, magnesium and copper.
» Used in Ayurvedic medicine to treat digestive and immune system diseases.
» Improves circulation and immunity.

- » Reduces pain.
- » Reduces susceptibility to infections, including SIBO, bacterial infections and colds.
- » Improves digestion and absorption of nutrients.
- » Provides electrolytes and trace elements for proper metabolic functions.
- » Helps prevent free radicals that can cause cognitive disorders such as Alzheimer's.
- » Relieves constipation, bloating, diarrhea and food sensitivities.
- » It has neuroprotective and chelating properties.
- » Binds and breaks down toxins in the body.
- » Repairs and protects the skin.
- » It contributes to the longevity of cells in the brain, heart, muscles and digestive tract.
- » Benefits in conditions such as gastritis, diarrhea, stomach ulcers, colitis and diabetes.
- » Stimulates bone growth.
- » Improves sleep quality and recovery after training.
- » It contributes to the rewiring of the brain and the elimination of negative neurons.
- » It has antibiotic properties
- » Optimizes mitochondrial functions.
- » Facilitates the absorption of nutrients and detoxifies the body.
- » Silica increases collagen synthesis.
- » It can act as a prebiotic and probiotic.

Properties:
- » Antioxidant
- » Antimicrobial
- » Antifungal
- » Antiviral
- » Anti-inflammatory
- » Anti-allergy

- » Antimutagenic
- » Antibiotic
- » Antispasmodic

- » Children: 13 drops, 3 times a day.
- » Young people and adults: 25 drops, 3 times a day.
- » You can take Humic/Fulvic with and without food.
- » For easy use, dilute it in water, soup/broth or your favorite beverage.
- » You can also add the drops directly to your food.
- » Humic/Fulvic is tasteless, odorless, does not affect the effectiveness of other supplements or medications, and does not require refrigeration.

PEKTICLEAN

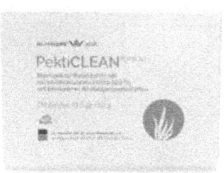

PektiClean® The import and export of molecules into and out of the cell is carried out through the plasma membrane.

The PektiClean® pectin molecule , on the other hand, can freely penetrate the cell membrane and bind contaminants directly there.

PektiClean® has a low molecular content of up to 60%, is negatively charged and unsaturated. This creates a strong attraction towards positively charged particles such as oxides or toxins. Therefore, the low molecular weight portion of PektiClean® It combines with toxins to produce a saturated compound. The saturated compound thus formed is excreted through the liver and kidneys. There is nothing else like it on the market. It takes out toxins and heavy metals from the whole body including the brain.

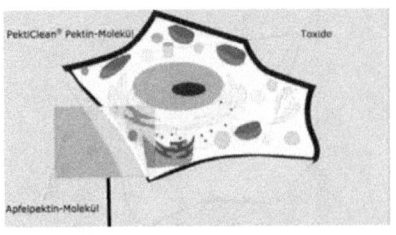

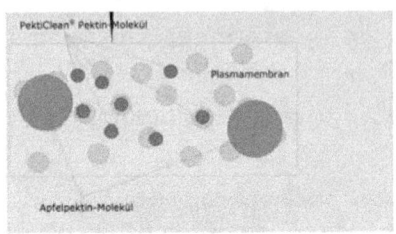

Mix the recommended dose of Pekticlean in 2 ounces/60ml of warm water or drink as a tea. You cannot eat anything one hour before or half an hour after taking Pekticlean. This supplement can be taken once or twice a day, or when the child is having a healing crisis, such as Herxheimer's symptoms.

In pounds	In kg	Dose
25 lb	11 kg	¼ of the envelope
50 lb	22 kg	½ of the envelope
100 lb	45 kg	1 full envelope

Chapter 8
Hyperbaric Oxygen Therapy (HBOT)

●Start-up Protocol
●Maintenance Protocol
●Benefits

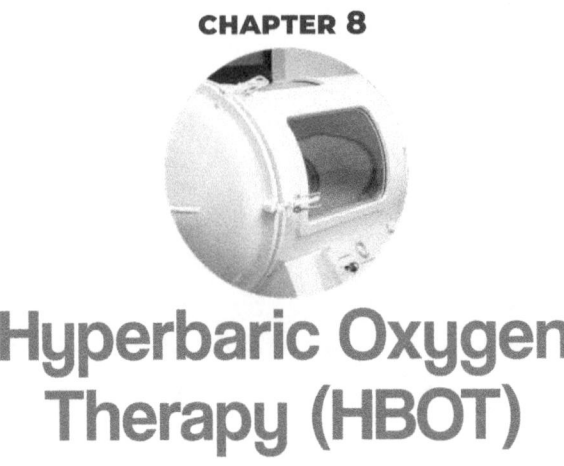

Hyperbaric Oxygen Therapy (HBOT)

This therapy is known as Hyperbaric Oxygen Therapy (HBOT) is the medical use of oxygen at pressures greater than atmospheric pressure.

The body needs oxygen to live, and the proper functioning of vital organs depends on it. The amount of oxygen that is assimilated depends largely on the atmospheric pressure, because the higher it is, the easier it is to breathe. The Earth's atmosphere normally exerts a pressure on its surface of 14.7 psi (pounds per inch) or 760 millimeters of mercury (mmHg) at sea level, this being equivalent to one atmosphere absolute (1 ATA). This atmosphere we breathe is a gaseous mixture (air) which is composed of approximately 21% oxygen and 79% nitrogen (and other things).

During the HBOT session the pressure inside the chamber increases two or three times the equivalent of atmospheric pressure, so you will breathe pure oxygen. With its partial pressure so drastically increased, oxygen permeates all the tissues of the body, and also causes the blood to be able to carry much more oxygen, since the blood plasma begins to transport the extra oxygen that the saturated hemoglobin can no longer carry.

Numerous studies have revealed that the use of hyperbaric oxygen in autoimmune disorders has been of great benefit. In the case of children with autism, there is evidence of encephalitis (inflammation of the brain) that may be caused by viral or bacterial infections, exposure to vaccines, or some other autoimmune process. Hyperbaric oxygen therapy also helps in conditions where intestinal disorders and problems with yeast and bacteria are present. There are improvements in speech, behavior, cognition, fine motor and gross motor, among other areas of improvement.

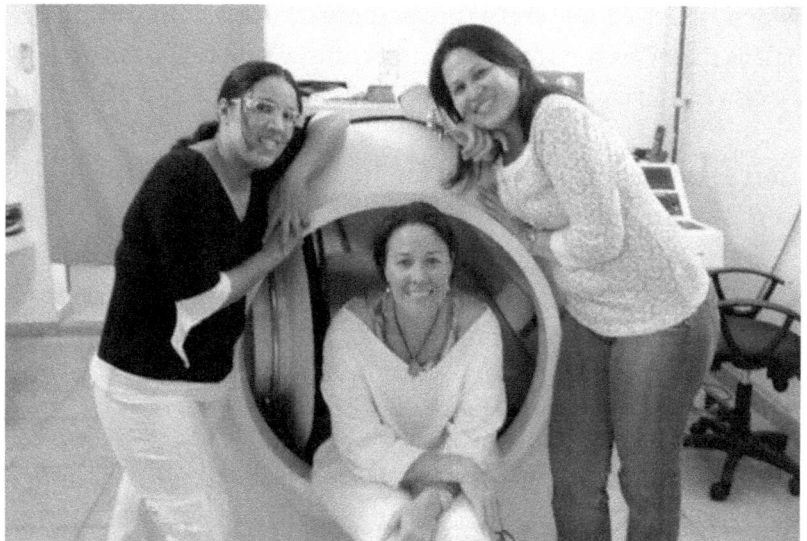

Lusmari Barroso, Kerri Rivera and Carolina Moreno at the Autism02 Clinic, Puerto Vallarta, Mexico - Year 2010

There are two treatment options for hyperbaric oxygen therapy for ASD:

INITIAL

Option 1: It consists of 40 sessions, 2 per day for 20 days each lasting 60 minutes at depth, with a pressurization of 1.75 ATA (atmosphere absolute). With this option we must do 2 sessions a day of 60 minutes each with a break of 4-8 hours between each session on the same day. The 60 minutes at 1.75ATA does not take into consideration the time for pressurization and decompression.

Option 2: This consists of 20 sessions, 1 per day ONLY. You can not do 2 sessions of 90 minutes at depth a day. There is too much oxidative stress from doing 2 of the 90-minute sessions in 1 day. The 90 minutes session are at a pressurization of 1.75 ATA (atmosphere absolute). The 90 minutes does not take into consideration the time to pressurize and to decompress.

MAINTENANCE

Once the initial phase is completed, it moves on to the maintenance phase, which is carried out every three months/90 days. In this phase, we do half as many sessions as we did in the initial phase. The maintenance phase also has two options:

Option 1: 20 sessions, 2 per day for 10 days of 60 minutes at depth at 1.75 ATA (atmosphere absolute)

Option 2: 10 sessions, 1 per day for 10 days of 90 minutes at depth at 1.75 ATA (atmosphere absolute)

THE TIME REQUIRED FOR THE HYPERBARIC CHAMBER TO PRESSURIZE AND DEPRESSURIZE DOES NOT COUNT AS A PART OF THE TIME AND SHOULD NOT BE CONSIDERED PART OF THE THERAPY TIME.

Benefits

- » Potential increase in cerebral perfusion.
- » Lowered intestinal and brain inflammation
- » Reduction of mitochondrial dysfunction.
- » Reduce irritability and sensory sensitivity
- » Improve muscle response.

Chapter 9
Complementary Supplements

- Probiotic
- GABA
- DMG
- L-Theanine
- 5-Hydroxytryptophan (5-HTP)
- Melatonin
- Taurine
- Omega-3
- Berberine
- Acetyl L-Carnitine

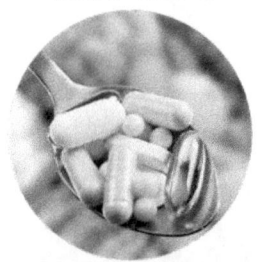

Complementary Supplements

The supplements described in this chapter are added between the breaks in parasite protocols or after the third Parasite Protocol has been completed. Depends on how the child is doing.

Ayurvedic Herbal Fermented Liquid Probiotic (email me kerri@kerririvera.com)

Those of you who have known me for years know that I stopped using probiotics around 2014. The reason was that I hadn't found a probiotic that really delivered on its promise of delivering live microorganisms to the gut. Most conventional probiotics are powders that are encapsulated in heartburn-resistant capsules. This not only affects digestion, but it also does not guarantee the probiotic's microorganisms survival rate. About 98% of them die due to the stomach acid. As a result, only less than 1 or 2% of the probiotics reach the intestine, which is insufficient to colonize. The worst thing is that anything that is marked as probiotic and is powder or powder in a capsule, is that they are not even probiotics, but they are PREbiotics. Prebiotics feed bacteria. You cannot pick and choose which bacteria will be fed. Will it be the friendly flora or the pathogenic flora like strep or staph. When you have ASD and/or PANDAS, the worst thing you can do is feed bacteria as is the case with the prebiotics. Therefore, if you use a traditional probiotic which is actually a prebiotic, your child will get worse.

On the other hand, AYURVEDIC FERMENTED HERBAL LIQUID PROBIOTIC is a liquid probiotic that uses a patented fermentation process with a pH similar to that of the stomach. This pH similarity between the probiotic and the stomach allows probiotic cultures to survive effectively during their transit to the intestines. As a pH-compatible liquid probiotic, it offers a beneficial way to administer live probiotic microorganisms and maintain proper intestinal health. It is a fermentation of the herbs of Ayurvedic medicine.

SEND ME AN EMAIL TO LET YOU KNOW WHERE TO GET IT KERRI@KERRIRIVERA.COM THIS TRUE PROBIOTIC DOES NOT FEED PATHOGENIC FLORA. I WILL STILL USE THIS LATER ON IF SOMEONE HAS PANDAS. IT IS PART OF THE HEALING THE GUT WHEN THE ATEC IS UNDER 15 OR NO MORE PANDAS SYMPTOMS ARE SEEN.

SUGGESTED DOSE

It is recommended to dilute the suggested dose in 1 of water or take it directly without diluting (as you prefer).

Age	Dose	Time
2 to 5 years	5 ml once a day	On an empty stomach or 15 minutes before a meal
6 to 9 years	15 ml once a day	On an empty stomach or 15 minutes before a meal
10 years and up	30 ml once a day	On an empty stomach or 15 minutes before a meal

GABA

It serves to fill the brain's receptor sites so that other messages cannot be transmitted, allowing for calm and relaxation. While GABA is an amino acid, it is classified as a neurotransmitter. It is the most abundant inhibitory neurotransmitter in the brain and can influence brain function.

Benefits:
- » Promotes relaxation of neurons
- » Can reduce seizures similar to Keppra.
- » Improves sleep
- » Reduces anxiety
- » Improves mood
- » Substantial language improvements
- » Focus
- » Concentration

Suggested schedule: On an empty stomach morning and night without food as much as possible.

Suggested Dose: Between 250mg and 2,500 mg - 2 times a day (Consult the dosage according to your case with Kerri)

DMG (DIMETHYLGLYCINE)

Is a non-protein amino acid present in plant and animal cells. DMG is considered a "methyl donor" or "methyl bank." In the body, with the help of a riboflavin coenzyme, DMG supplies methyl groups that bind to folic acid to form methylene tetrahydrofolate, an important component of many biochemical processes in the body, including cellular perception and response. Also involved in maintaining healthy homocysteine levels.

Benefits:

- » Immune system support
- » Support brain and cognitive function
- » Improved liver function.
- » Improvement with speech focus and concentrations.
- » Modulation of the nervous system

Suggested schedule: On an empty stomach once a day. If the child is taking GABA, both supplements can be given at the same time.

Single Dose: 900 mg on an empty stomach in the morning before noon all together. You can start with 125 mg and go up by 125 mg a day till you reach the maximum dose of

L-THEANINE

It is a non-protein amino acid found mainly in tea leaves, especially green tea. It acts as a neurological modulator and promotes positive changes in the brain, increasing the production of neurotransmitters such as serotonin and dopamine, which are involved in the regulation of mood and cognitive function. Additionally, L-theanine has been observed to stimulate alpha brain waves, associated with relaxation and attention. These properties may contribute to its beneficial effects on stress reduction, mood improvement, concentration, and focus.

Suggested schedule: On an empty stomach two or three times a day with GABA and DMG.

Suggested dose: 250 mg capsule

- » Less than 5 years: ½ capsule 2 to 3 times a day.
- » Over 5 years: 1 capsule 2 to 3 times a day
- » Can take 2 to 3 capsules 3 times a day if better because of it.

ACETYL L-CARNITINE

Research indicates that acetyl L-carnitine can help children with autism in many ways. The most important benefit is an improvement in the child's behavior. It can also improve language skills, improve nervous system function, and muscle tone.

Recommended doses: For children, 250 mg to 500 mg three times a day, and for adolescents and adults it can be upwards of 1,500 mg three times a day. Acetyl L-carnitine is ideally taken without food and can be given with GABA, DMG etc.

5-HYDROXYTRYPTOPHAN (5-HTP)

Although the human body naturally produces 5-hydroxytryptophan (5-HTP) from tryptophan, there are cases in which 5-HTP levels may be insufficient to meet the body's needs. Additionally, some people may have difficulty properly synthesizing or absorbing tryptophan, which can result in lower levels of 5-HTP and serotonin.

Benefits:
  » Mood improvement
  » Anxiety reduction
  » Sleep improvement
  » Appetite control
  » Relief of migraine symptoms

Suggested Schedule: 3 times a day in 4-hour intervals and can be consumed with or without food.

When there is anxiety, it helps a lot.

Suggested dose: Between 50 mg and 150 mg - 3 times a day.

MELATONIN

Is a natural hormone that is produced in the pineal gland of the brain. It plays a crucial role in regulating the sleep-wake cycle and is closely related to the body's circadian rhythm. Low levels of melatonin are considered a very common cause of insomnia.

Several double-blind studies have shown that melatonin supplementation is effective in promoting sleep when melatonin levels are low. However, if a person takes melatonin when their levels are balanced, nothing happens.

For people with glutathione deficiency, melatonin is important because it stimulates the production of glutathione peroxidase.

Beneficits:
- » Sleep improvement
- » Circadian rhythm regulation
- » Antioxidant effect
- » Anti-inflammatory properties

Suggested time: 1 hour before bed

For melatonin to have an optimal effect, it is recommended to take it in a dark or low-light environment. This is because the body's natural production of melatonin is influenced by light exposure. The pineal gland in the brain begins to secrete melatonin in response to decreased ambient light. Under normal conditions, as night approaches and light decreases, melatonin production increases, which helps prepare the body for sleep. Exposure to bright light sources, such as screens of electronic devices, should also be avoided before going to bed, as bright light can inhibit melatonin production and affect sleep quality.

Suggested Dose: Up to 15 mg daily (If your child takes GABA, you can take both supplements together in the evening).

TAURINE

It plays a calming role as a neurotransmitter by counteracting the stimulating effect of glutamate. It also has a very important antioxidant function in white blood cells, leukocytes, and lymphocytes. These cells are important in protecting the body from foreign substances and invading organisms. It is a neuro protector.

The formation of tauro-cholic acid, a key component of bile, requires L-taurine. Bile allows the absorption of fat-soluble vitamins A, D, E and K, as well as essential fatty acids.

Benefits:
- » Antioxidant protection from free radicals.
- » Support for people suffering from seizures.
- » Promotes neurogenesis and synaptogenesis.

Suggested schedule: 2 times a day without food, can go with GABA and DMG

Suggested dose:
- » 250 mg up to 2,000 mg (2 times a day)
- » (Consult the dosage according to your case with Kerri)

OMEGA-3

Omega-3 fatty acids are important for normal brain function, cardiovascular health, and neurological health. They reduce brain inflammation which is beneficial for speech. They are especially important in the roles during the developing baby's brain.

Suggested Schedule: With food in the morning and/or mid day.

Dose:
- » 25 lb: 1 capsule
- » 50 lb: 2 capsules
- » 75 lb: 3 capsules
- » 100 lb: 4 capsules

BERBERINE

It has been studied for its beneficial health properties, including its ability to protect neurons. Berberine exhibits neuroprotective effects by reducing oxidative stress and inflammation in the brain, which may help prevent cellular damage and promote nerve cell survival. In addition, berberine has been observed to regulate the expression of genes and proteins related to neuronal growth and survival.

Berberine is an anti depressant, anti cancer, anti infection, anti fatty liver, anti-inflammatory etc. Berberine is also anti-parasitic, antiviral, antibacterial, and antifungal. It helps destroy biofilm and does not allow the replication of pathogenic bacteria. Berberine does not damage the intestinal flora. It helps in sealing leaky gut which is very important for healing the body and problems with allergies. It also helps with appetite. Many parents say that their children always want to eat more and more. Berberine helps. More importantly for PANDAS, the berberine helps to keep the bacteria from hijacking the cells. This is VERY important as you can imagine. Once bacteria get into the cells. It is very difficult to get them out. The bacteria can stay hidden and come out later like during puberty.

Benefits:
- » Antibacterial
- » Antifungal/candida, attacks the cell wall of the candida/yeast/fungus
- » Antivirus

149

- » Antimicrobial
- » Anti-inflammatory
- » Antiparasitic
- » Anti-aging
- » Antidepressant
- » Antioxidant
- » Antihistamine
- » Anti-cancer
- » Against dementia
- » Anti-MRSA
- » Reduces oxidative stress
- » Inhibits intracellular invasion and cell sequestration.
- » Inhibits the formation of biofilms.
- » Inhibits intestinal infections
- » Intestinal antimicrobial
- » Treats alterations in the intestinal microbiome, such as intestinal dysbiosis and bacterial imbalances.
- » Increases intestinal health
- » Increases heart health
- » Reduces high blood pressure
- » Eradicates the infection
- » Lowers blood sugar.
- » Reduces LDL/bad cholesterol
- » Increases healthy HDL/cholesterol
- » Reduces belly fat
- » Reduces insulin resistance.
- » Helps with weight loss.
- » Balances leptin levels to help you not feel so hungry
- » Helps in cases of neurodegenerative diseases.
- » SIBO, which is the number one cause of IBS/irritable bowel syndrome, as good or better than ABX/rifaximin
- » Improved liver function
- » Reduces liver inflammation.
- » Treats nonalcoholic fatty liver disease
- » Seals leaky gut/tightens joints in gut
- » Normalizes appetite

» Regulates blood glucose.

» Reduces fasting glucose

» Balances lipids

» Relaxes stress

» PCOS, polycystic ovary syndrome; acne, dysmenorrhea, infertility, baldness, insulin resistance, sleep apnea, glucose disturbance, cardiovascular diseases, type 2 diabetes, triglycerides, depression and obesity.

Suggested schedule: With food, 30 minutes before meals, during or after meals.

Dose: 500 mg to 3,000 mg per day divided between meals. The standard dose is 500 mg 3 times a day.

IODINE

Iodine has been recognized as an effective broad-spectrum bactericide and is also effective against yeasts, molds, fungi, viruses, and protozoa. It is also helpful for hypothyroidism which many of the children on the ASD have. TSH is an important marker for diagnosing hypothyroidism. If the TSH is between .60 and 1.50 all is well. Over 1.50 begins hypothyroidism. You would be so surprised to hear what doctors tell us. Like 4.65 TSH is "normal". The person is lethargic and can't focus. But they are fine. Imagine?!

Lugol's iodine, iodine in general, is liquid. You can add the drops of the iodine to a glass of water in the morning. Lugol's iodine is the preference of those who know iodine well. It is taken between 2 drops and 40 drops once a day depending on age, weight and issues.

Chapter 10
What to do if my child gets sick?

- Fever
- Flu, Cough, Nasal Congestion
- Nebulizations with Structured Silver
- Earache
- Sores and Skin Rashes
- Sore Throat
- Dental and Oral Pains

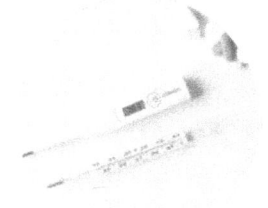

What to do if my child gets sick?

 Fever

It has long been recognized as an important tool in the healing process. The process of warming the body is called "hyperthermia." Hyperthermia or a run-of-the-mill fever can be very effective against cancer cells, various pathogens, or invading organisms that cannot "tolerate heat." Hyperthermia may not kill any pathogens in the body, but it may reduce the number of invaders in the body to a manageable level for the immune system. Hyperthermia may also be responsible for stimulating the immune system to produce cytokines, the production of antibodies and the release of toxins.

In practice, if your child develops a fever, it is not an error in the body that needs to be corrected, it is a mechanism that brings the body closer to healing. Instead of administering acetaminophen/paracetamol or some other fever-reducing remedy, apply a wet cloth to your forehead and neck, and let your body do its job. We can also give a hot bath then when we get out, the contrast helps to reduce the fever. We must always be vigilant, that the temperature does not rise too much or too quickly to cause seizures, we must use common sense and trust our instincts. In case they have to give medications to reduce fever, the indicated is ibuprofen never paracetamol.

Paracetamol reduces intracellular levels of glutathione. Glutathione is the body's antioxidant that is much needed in times of fever.

In case you must give fever-reducing medication, ibuprofen (never paracetamol) is indicated.

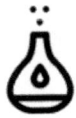 ## Flu, Cough, and Nasal Congestion

Humidifier with CD: For every liter of water add 9 drops of CD in the humidifier and place in the room where the child sleeps.

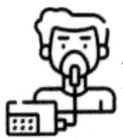 ## Nebulizations with Structured Silver

Fill the reservoir of the nebulizer with structured silver. No need to dilute with saline solution. Turn on the nebulizer and inhale until all the liquid in the reservoir is gone. You can do as many hours as the child will tolerate sitting with the nebulizer mask on. This procedure can be done all day and night or as many hours as one tolerates. There are people who do it all night while they sleep.

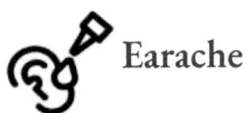 ## Earache

2 activated drops of CD in 30ml of water.

Lie on your side, fill the ear with the liquid and pull the ear so that the liquid enters the ear well. Do this procedure every hour until the pain subsides. If the pain is very acute, repeat the procedure every 15 minutes.

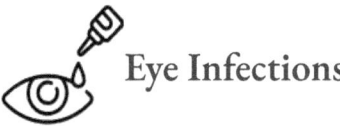 # Eye Infections

1 activated drop of CD in 60ml of water.

Apply 2 or 3 drops every hour until you see improvements.

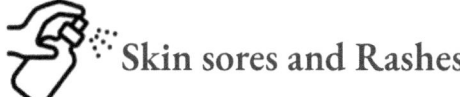 # Skin sores and Rashes

For every 30ml/1oz of water, 20 activated drops of CD. Spray the affected region or apply gently with fingers. Do this 4 times a day minimum or every hour if necessary.

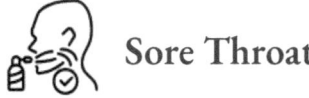 # Sore Throat

20 drops per 30ml/1oz of water, use a spray bottle.

Spray liberally on the affected area every 15-60 minutes all day long until gone.

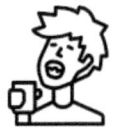 # Dental and Oral Pain

Prepare a dose of 10 activated drops in half a glass of water: gargle every two hours until the tooth pain disappears and then twice a day until the mouth and gums are completely healthy. If there are cavities, it will be necessary to go to the dentist. It is a good idea to add DMSO to the water so that the CD absorbs into the tissue in the mouth better.

Chapter 11
Frequently asked questions and answers

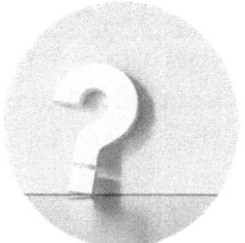

Frequently asked questions and answers

1.— QUESTION: My son loves juices and soft drinks. Can I give him sugar-free soft drinks from time to time to satisfy his craving?

ANSWER: No, never! You can make hibiscus tea and dilute it with more water so that the color of the tea/water comes out more pink and less dark burgundy. Stevia or monk fruit is added to this tea/water to make it sweet like juice or soft drinks.

2.— QUESTION: My son does not have autism, he "just" has ADHD, what is the protocol for these cases?

ANSWER: "Just" doesn't mean ADHD isn't a big problem. So, you use your ATEC, and every 90 days do the ATEC until it reaches 0. Meanwhile, you should do the full protocol as it is written with diet and everything until the ATEC is at 0 and you no longer have any ADHD/spectrum autistic.

3.— QUESTION: For a 4-year-old child with normal to watery stools, who does NOT have constipation, can magnesium citrate be given? Or should it be magnesium glycinate?

ANSWER: We use magnesium glycinate for those who have normal and formed stools or those who have had diarrhea in their past or currently.

4.— QUESTION: My 19-year-old daughter who has a lot of difficulty sleeping and nightmares who takes medication for this. I was supplementing with melatonin, but they told me that it was addictive and that if she continued doing so, her body could stop producing melatonin. Is that true? I had to give in to the medication because neither she nor I could sleep.

ANSWER: Not true at all. Melatonin does not cause addiction. There are even studies of the benefits of high doses of melatonin. Pharmaceutical medications do cause dependency, however.

5.— QUESTION: Is it good to give L-GLUTAMINE to a child who has a low glutamate diet? Are glutamate and L-GLUTAMINE the same thing?

ANSWER: It is not the same. Giving l-glutamine to a child on the ASD is like throwing gasoline on a fire. Glutamate is formed directly from glutamine by deamidation via phosphate-activated glutaminase, a reaction that also produces ammonia. Glutamate plays key roles in linking carbohydrate and amino acid metabolism through the tricarboxylic acid (TCA) cycle, as well as nitrogen trafficking and ammonia homeostasis in the brain. Avoid at all costs.

6.— QUESTION: We are doing the low glutamate diet and I wanted to know if the rice can be normal, or does it have to be gluten-free?

ANSWER: All types of rice are gluten-free. Try adding fats like MCT/C8 to your rice so the child consumes less carbohydrates/rice. The fat will make the child fuller faster.

7.— QUESTION: Can we give buckwheat since it does not have gluten?

ANSWER: Buckwheat cannot be used. Even though it is gluten-free, it does have glutamate. This glutamate damages the brain and its neurons. Glutamate damages the blood brain barrier allowing for more and more toxins to get into the brain. And, on the other hand, it is extremely high in carbohydrates. In the body, carbohydrates are sugars. Sugar feeds candida and parasites as well as causing inflammation in the body.

8.— QUESTION: I can't find Mebendazole in Ecuador, what can I replace it with?

ANSWER: There is nothing like mebendazole. Mebendazole is an anti-parasitic medication that does not damage the intestinal flora, does not kill other pathogens, and does not pass through the liver. It only kills parasites and leaves the intestine in 12 hours. Try to get mebendazole.

9.— QUESTION: My daughter is on a low-glutamate diet, but the only thing I haven't been able to take away from her is almond milk. Any recommendations for one she can take?

ANSWER: It is not necessary to drink any type of milk, even nut milks. But, if she doesn't like water, you can give her coconut milk. If she does not like the taste of the coconut milk. You can begin reducing the almond milk with coconut milk over a period of a week till she is drinking all coconut milk. It is done by starting with 7oz almond milk with 1oz coconut milk. Every day, swap out 1oz of the almond milk which we cannot drink because of the high glutamate and replace it with 1oz of coconut. We do this for 8 days till there is 0 almond milk and only 8oz of coconut milk.

10.— QUESTION: I am transitioning to the carnivore diet and I notice my son is very irritable.

ANSWER: It is not uncommon to be like this when you switch from a high carbohydrate diet to a no carbohydrate diet. A high carbohydrate diet is unhealthy for many reasons. Primarily, a high carbohydrate diet feeds candida and parasites. On the other hand, a diet high in carbohydrates causes inflammation in the body. It is not harmful. Yet it can be uncomfortable. You can make the transition over a few weeks if the prior diet had been very high in carbohydrates and/or processed foods. Berberine also helps to control the glucose levels. You can add one capsule per meal at this point.

11.— QUESTION: What do you recommend in case of the flu?

ANSWER: It all depends on whether the child stops eating or not. If they do not stop eating, everything remains the same and we add the structured silver to the nebulizer and inhale as many hours as possible. If the child stops eating, we must stop everything. We only make CD baths and CD in the humidifier. We can do nebulized structured silver and 5 ml of structured silver orally every hour. You should also give a pedialyte-type electrolyte beverage. It is best to get one without coloring added. Usually, the coconut flavored one does not have added colors. If you start to worry a lot. The medicine that does not affect children negatively is ibuprofen. Those fever reducers that are not good for children are Tylenol and acetaminophen/paracetamol.

12.— QUESTION: If the child is to receive 26 drops according to their weight, but only tolerates 15, can we start the PP at that dose?

ANSWER: If the child cannot tolerate more than 15 drops when his full dose according to his weight is 26 drops and he is taking all of the other supplements in the protocol then he can start the PP.

13.— QUESTION: Can BSO (black seed oil) be used on food?

ANSWER: It is not recommended to add it to foods since it has a very strong flavor. It is best to mix it with the "chondroitin/oleic acid/D" product because of its pleasant flavor. Can be given together in a syringe during meals and chased down with water.

14.— QUESTION: My son eat every 4 hours, what happens if I can't get in all of the CD doses.

ANSWER: CD doses are given every 45 minutes. It has nothing to do with food. For example, if your child will eat at 4pm and the next dose at 4:10pm, give the dose at 3:55pm and feed at 4pm.

15.— QUESTION: Is allulose allowed?

ANSWER: Yes.

16.— QUESTION: How do I know which magnesium is indicated for my child?

ANSWER: If your child has had or has constipation, we use magnesium citrate. But, if your child has or has had diarrhea, loose stools, or normally formed stools, we use magnesium glycinate.

17.— QUESTION: My son was diagnosed with autism. Where should I start?

ANSWER: Immediately do the ATEC score at www.autism.org and start the low glutamate or carnivore diet. I have 2 diet options. Whichever you feel that you will be able to follow at this point in time. Start my protocol with social media groups, my new book or make an appointment with me. Never lose time. We must get going as soon as we hear those words. That gives us the best chance for full recovery.

18.— QUESTION: How can I know what diet is best for my child?

ANSWER: You must look and see what he likes to eat now. If your child eats a lot of carbohydrates. The first step is to take out the foods that are not allowed in the diet. If your child likes chicken and meats, you can immediately try the carnivore diet.

19.— QUESTION: We started the carnivore diet, and my son has diarrhea. Is it normal?

ANSWER: It is not uncommon. We can use bentonite clay orally in water 2 to 3 times a day in water to reduce the frequency of the diarrhea. The diarrhea does not usually last more than 6 to 8 weeks. This is a sign that the intestine is healing.

20.— QUESTION: How do I calculate the amount of fat my child should consume at each meal on a ketogenic or carnivore diet?

ANSWER: Normally, we think about 6 tablespoons a day or 50% of calories from fat is best.

21.— QUESTION: Can excess animal protein damage the kidneys?

ANSWER: You remember that there is a lot of propaganda on the internet. Also, in social media groups. I direct you to read Dr. Shawn Baker's book or to visit Dr. Robert Kiltz's website www.doctorkiltz.com for further confirmation of the health benefits of the carnivore diet versus the propaganda. Humans were carnivores for millions of years. It has always been our native diet.

22.— QUESTION: What is the recommended time to follow a carnivore diet?

ANSWER: There are people who do it for life, decades. But it would be good to do it until at least the ATEC gets as low as possible and as close to 0 as possible if not all the way to 0.

23.— QUESTION: Can I use coconut oil on a carnivore diet?

ANSWER: In autism recovery, it is possible. MCT/C8 is easy to use because it has no taste or odor. But animal fats are the fats for the carnivore diet. We are not so worried about this. The important thing is a diet with high fat, moderate protein and low to zero carbohydrates. But a carnivore purist would say no. For our purposes for healing autism, MCT/C8 is fine.

24.— QUESTION: How many carbohydrates are allowed on the low glutamate diet that my child can consume at each meal?

ANSWER: It is important to do as few carbohydrates as possible when trying to heal the gut/brain/body. I feel that 25 to 50 carbs a day is a maximum. BUT there are children who are almost vegan and consume between 300 and 500 carbohydrates a day. It's a problem. But, little by little, we add more fats like MCT/C8 to your carbohydrates like rice or potato, which you will crave less and less of as you increase the fats. Increasing fat to the diet helps to drive down the carb cravings.

25: QUESTION: How can I meet the requirements of vitamins and minerals if fruit consumption is restricted?

ANSWER: Well, if you're thinking that this is how we survived for the past 3 million years that humans have been on the planet and it wasn't. Think about the eskimos/Inuk like Nanook of the North in the Canadian Arctic. They have never seen a fruit or vegetable in their lives nor have their ancestors and they don't need them at all. Vitamins and minerals come from red, fatty meats. I use Humic/Fulvic for everyone to get the 75+ minerals and electrolytes for the best of health and healing.

26.— QUESTION: My son started the low carbohydrate diet and is losing weight. What should I do?

ANSWER: Always weigh your child every 30 days, first thing in the morning, without clothes and without a meal. If he loses weight, you will realize that you are not giving him the necessary amount of fat and calories that he needs. It is very important to pay attention to the amount of calories that the children are consuming. Never go below the number of calories for the age of the child.

27.— QUESTION: My son does not like to eat animal protein. What can I do to ensure you get all the necessary macronutrients in your diet?

ANSWER: A high carbohydrate diet is not ideal for healing a damaged gut and compromised system. In the case of children with ASD, it is important to lower carbohydrates, which are sugars in the body, and increase the fats and proteins. If you think it is impossible at this time to switch from a diet high in carbohydrates to a diet high in fat and protein. Start the complete protocol and see if in a few months the child is more flexible because they are improving from the rest of the protocol. Little by little we can introduce animal proteins and animal fats and exclude carbohydrates.

28.— QUESTION: Why are bone broths not recommended?

ANSWER: Because when you cook the bones for a long time, as is the case with bone broth, it draws out the glutamate. Glutamate is very bad for the brain. It also causes behavioral issues.

29.— QUESTION: We are vegans. What options do we have regarding nutrition for my child with autism?

ANSWER: For vegans, I use more MCT/C8 with each food. For example, if you eat quinoa, rice, potatoes, grains, cereals etc that are carbohydrates. It is important to add 2 to 3 tablespoons of MCT/C8 on top of these foods. If the child tolerates avocados. It is possible to give several avocados a day. You can even give an avocado as a snack with 1 spoon of MCT/C8 mixed inside like guacamole. Anyway, try to be vegan with high fats. That would be the first step towards making an unhealthy diet, healthier.

30.— QUESTION: Why do you use CD and not CDS for autism?

ANSWER: Since 2010, when I started using chlorine dioxide (CD/MMS) there was no such thing as CDS. Andreas Kalcker spoke to a group of us like Jim Humble and others in the movement in Prague about CDS in January 2012. Since 2010, children have been recovering from autism with CD/MMS. It works and there is no reason to fix something which is not broken. However, in September of 2012, I decided to try CDS with 60 families who were using CD successfully but were interested in trying it. We made the change from whatever amount of CD drops we were taking to the same number of milliliters of CDS. That is, if the person was taking 20 drops of CD a day. They switched to 20 ml CDS a day. Within a few days, all the families began to say that they were seeing regression in many areas where they have previously improved. Many parents were begging me to return to CD. I also saw regression with my own son regarding his sleep. But I decided to continue with the CDS for a while longer even though everyone else had gone back to CD. Each day increased by 1 ml more until he could sleep as well as he did when he took the CD. By the time we reached 120 ml of CDS when his prior full dose of CD was 70 drops, and it still wasn't enough. The flavor was VERY strong by the time we reached 120 ml CDS. In the case of ASD, CD is superior for recovery and works far better than CDS. My experience with 100,000+ children since 2010 has been that the results with CD are superior to CDS. If one feels like using CDS. Give it a try. Use your ATEC every 90 days. If it doesn't go down or if it doesn't go down very fast, consider switching to CD. Chlorine dioxide is very noble. So, whether you use CD or CDS there will be benefits.

It has been my experience that the ability to get to the ATEC of 0 most efficiently is with CD.

31.— QUESTION. If I have CD left over from the previous day, should I throw it away or can I use it up the next day?

ANSWER: Put the bottle in the refrigerator overnight. The next day you can continue using it. Typically, a bottle can last in the refrigerator up to 1 to 3 days.

32.— QUESTION: Should I keep the CD bottle with the day's doses in the refrigerator? I don't like cold drinks, what can I do?

ANSWER: It is not necessary to keep the bottle in the refrigerator. Just don't leave it near windows where the sun shines in. The sun weakens the CD.

33.— QUESTION: My child spends more than 5 hours at school, and I cannot complete the 16 doses, does this affect the protocol?

ANSWER: Unfortunately, when we do not achieve 16+ CD doses a day, it does affect the results. We can send the structured silver to the school in a "PBA free" plastic bottle. But it is not the same as CD doses. I'm sorry. The magic is in the frequency of the dosing. I have seen families give 8 double doses instead of 16 normal doses. Is not the same. The CD only lasts for 45 minutes in the body. You must keep pressure on the pathogens all day. That is why 16 or more doses is what gets the child better faster. Out of a 24-hour day we must try to give more hours of doses then we do giving the pathogens a chance to thrive and survive.

34.— QUESTION: How many minutes should I wait to give a dose of CD after each meal?

ANSWER: The CD doses are every 45 minutes. If you are going to start eating at 4pm, give your CD dose at 3:55pm. If your meal starts at 4:30pm and the child is still eating.

It would be good to give 5 minutes after finishing the meal. We do not want to lose the rhythm of dosing every 45 minutes.

35.— QUESTION: Can I add apple juice or non-dairy milk to disguise the taste of the CD?

ANSWER: When you put CD in milk of any type, it cancels out the CD. And the question of juices is a big one. Juice has a LOT of carbohydrates which are sugars in the body. Sugars in the body feed pathogens like candida and parasites. Sugars also cause inflammation in the body. After this juice problem, most also have many antioxidants that cancel out CD. It is preferable to dilute the CD in more water for each intake or buy a sweetener called SWEETLEAF (brand) Stevia. This product does not affect the potential of the CD and is not sugar. It is a natural sweetener.

36.— QUESTION: Since my son started taking CD, his teeth turned yellow. What is causing this and how can I fix it?

ANSWER: There is a biofilm on the teeth. CD kills biofilm. Biofilm has virus, bacteria, candida, parasites, and heavy metals. It is a very good thing to remove biofilm from the body, including what is on the teeth. It removes the discoloration on its own. If the color bothers you a lot. You can go to the dentist for a dental cleaning. That will get rid of it. Of course, it will go away by itself at some point in the near future.

37.— QUESTION: My child wants to eat things that are not edible, like dirt, crayons, paper, and soap. Why is this?

ANSWER: It is called PICA, and it is a symptom of the presence of parasites in the body. It goes away as the parasite load in the body goes down.

38.— QUESTION: My Son likes to eat salt, sometimes I have to hide the saltshaker, why this desire to eat salt?

ANSWER: One of the biomarkers of autism has to do with a deficiency in fatty acid processing and delta 6 desaturase. People with autism cannot develop immune mediators as healthy people normally do. The gut biome compensates for this by producing an unusually high amount of propionic acid which is used as an immune mediator. In a study where mice were injected with propionic acid, the mice developed self-inflammation/brain swelling, just as occurs in people with autism. They were able to recover the mice by feeding them salt, which has a neutralizing effect on propionic acid. This is why people with autism crave salt. The body is trying to heal itself.

39.— QUESTION: Do you recommend diatomaceous earth as part of the deworming process?

ANSWER: In 2012, when the parasite protocol came out, there were many products involved. Some of them like mebendazole, castor oil and chanka piedras/stone breaker are still necessary and very good. Others were not so good. Among those that were not good is oral diatomaceous earth (DE). There were 2 problems. One problem was that those who had suffered with constipation had more problems with constipation. And the worst thing for everyone was that the diatomaceous earth (DE) shredded the parasites. This shredding of the parasites released more toxicity into the body than if the parasites died with mebendazole and came out intact. More problems with unwanted behavior, among other setbacks due to the higher level of toxicity. H7 helps a lot with the toxins from the parasites. So does pekticlean. I still prefer a cleaner and less toxic parasite kill without DE.

40.— QUESTION: My son is prescribed 25 mg of mebendazole, but I can only find 100 mg pills. How can I calculate the dosage?

ANSWER: With a knife, split the 100mg tablet into 4 equal parts. Each part has 25mg. You can give him a quarter of the tablet 2 times a day and save the other 2 leftovers for the next day. You can crush the tablet with a spoon for administering with other supplements or in a beverage.

41.— QUESTION: Why is seawater no longer used?

ANSWER: There was a time when I used it. But, after finding HUMIC/FULVIC that is so much better. I switched to HUMIC/FULVIC back in 2016. The list of what the HUMIC/FULVIC does is very long. It's elsewhere in this book. When I see that there is something better, safer, and less expensive. I change. In the case of HUMIC/FULVIC and seawater this was the case. HUMIC/FULVIC is safer because it comes from deep in the earth away from toxins like radiation, among other unwanted things. Toxins from humanity cannot reach it. About 50% of children with ASD have diarrhea. When you have diarrhea, you lose minerals. When you lose minerals, we must add more. Seawater causes diarrhea for many, especially those who are prone to diarrhea. When we gave more seawater to someone with diarrhea, it would only make things worse. So, it is very difficult to give more seawater to a person who already has diarrhea. HUMIC/FULVIC does not cause diarrhea nor constipation. However, the list of benefits from HUMIC/FULVIC is what convinced me to switch over. It is worth repeating here its benefits above 75+ minerals and electrolytes, HUMIC/FULVIC is a very small molecule that is bioavailable in the body.

» It comes from deep within the earth and is organic.
» Regulates the bioavailability of iron, calcium, magnesium and copper.
» Comes from Ayurvedic medicine and it was used to treat digestive diseases as well as the immune system.
» Improves circulation and immunity.
» Reduces pain
» Reduces susceptibility to infection.
» SIBO
» UTIs
» Bacterial infections
» Colds
» Improves digestion and absorption of nutrients.

- » Electrolytes and trace elements for proper metabolic functions
- » Helps prevent free radicals that cause cognitive disorders such as Alzheimer's.
- » Relieves constipation, bloating, diarrhea and food sensitivities.
- » Neuro protector
- » Chelates out heavy metals from the brain.
- » Binds and breaks down toxins.
- » Repairs and protects the skin
- » May prevent colon cancer
- » Extends the life of cells in the brain, heart, muscles, digestive tract.
- » Gastritis, diarrhea, stomach ulcers, colitis, diabetes
- » Stimulates bone growth
- » Improves sleep
- » Sports training recovery
- » Eliminates stress
- » Rewires the brain, eliminates negative neurons.
- » Antibiotic
- » Kills malaria
- » Antipsychotic
- » Optimize mitochondria
- » Helps absorb nutrients.
- » Detoxes the body
- » Silica increases collagen synthesis
- » Prebiotic/probiotic
- » It attracts free radicals and eliminates them, as well as it does with heavy metals.

42.— QUESTION: What should I do in cases of vomiting?

ANSWER: Change what you are doing. There are many possibilities as to why one vomits. It is possible that there is a stomach virus or bacteria. It is possible that some food you ate was bad for you.

Giving too many doses of CD without eating for a long period of time. It is possible that you gave the child more CD than he tolerates and might have to consider reducing the drops in the 16 doses.

43.— QUESTION: What to do when children have the flu?

ANSWER: It all depends on whether the child stops eating or not. If he stops eating all together then we only do CD baths, nebulized structured silver, HUMIC/FULVIC, and should take pedialyte without dyes. If they continue eating, then we can continue with the full protocol.

44.— QUESTION: Which supplements can be given with food, and which should be taken on an empty stomach?

ANSWER: Almost everything can go with food. Those that should go without food are: CD, structured silver, GABA, DMG, Pekticlean, and H7.

45.— QUESTION: Can I mix some supplements to facilitate the routine effectively?

ANSWER: Of course! All the supplements other than those that do NOT go with food can go together with food.

46.— QUESTION: Are colloidal silver and structured silver the same thing?

ANSWER: They are not the same and one should not use oral colloidal silver. Structured silver is alkaline, it works with the immune system, it does not leave the structure and 99% of the structured silver leaves the body in under 24 hours. It does not damage the intestinal flora. Colloidal silver is acidic, not everything comes out of the body, and it can damage the good flora. Please see the structured silver section of the book on page 92

47.— QUESTION: My son has yellow palms and soles of his feet. Why is this happening and what can I do to help?

ANSWER: It is an indication of free heavy metals in the body. It is a good sign. This is to say that if we use bentonite baths, oral chelators such as EDTA and zeolite that they will take the heavy metals out of the body. The toxic heavy metals are now just waiting for a chelator to take them out of the body. They are no longer attached to biofilms nor organs or bones. CD is good at neutralizing heavy metals of their charge. When the CD neutralizes the charge from the heavy metal, it is easier to remove them with oral and bath chelators.

48.— QUESTION: Does this protocol have any side effects?

ANSWER: NO! First of all, a side effect is something that can happen from medications that come from the pharmacy. All pharmaceutical medications can have side effects. In the case of CD and the CD protocol there are no side effects. It is possible to have a Herxheimer reaction. A Herxheimer reaction is when we kill pathogens faster than the body can take out the toxins. For this reason, I use supplements that help the body remove toxins from the body such as H7, Pekticlean and ultra binder. A Herxheimer is neither dangerous nor permanent. I have seen with a simple change from a junk food diet to a clean diet that the person had a Herxheimer's reaction. This protocol has been in use in parts since 2010 with me in ASD cases. I have never seen anyone hurt or have any permanent negative effect.

49: QUESTION: What do I use for toothpaste and mouthwash?

ANSWER: Everyday chlorine dioxide (ClO2) products such as toothpaste, mouthwash, among others, exist because of the great scientist Howard Alliger.

Howard Alliger was a pioneer in the field of chlorine dioxide and first discovered its healing properties in the 1970s. Prior to this time, ClO2 was known as a disinfecting, bleaching and descaling agent, used in large scale applications such as disinfection of municipal water supplies and bleaching of paper and pulp. But, at that time, chlorine dioxide, being a gas, was not transportable or available for personal use. Determined to find a way to use chlorine dioxide itself, Howard developed a method to manufacture the compound on the laboratory bench and into a form suitable for use in the body. While experimenting, he even used chlorine dioxide on his own cuts and infections and found that they healed surprisingly quickly. He then patented his method of producing chlorine dioxide in 1978 and developed stable products incorporating this technology, which today are available to improve our health in many ways. Howard's efforts opened the field of chlorine dioxide for personal care and today there are hundreds of patents on chlorine dioxide. Howard founded Frontier Pharmaceutical, Inc. in 1993, where he and his daughter Valerie worked together for more than 20 years. Valerie continues to run the company to carry on her father's legacy. To see all of Frontier's amazing products, visit

https://frontierpharm.com/kerri

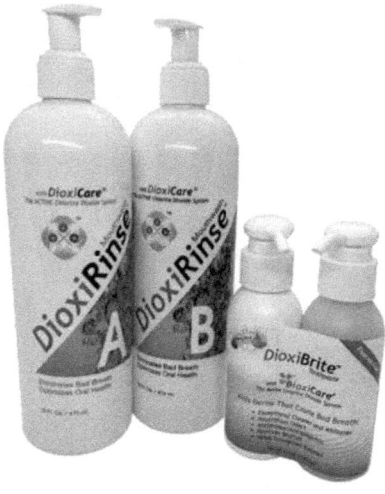

Chapter 12
Jim Humble
A Legacy of Hope and a Light in the Darkness

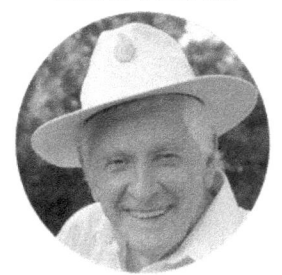

Jim Humble
A Legacy of Hope and a Light in the Darkness

Rest in peace great friend, teacher, humanitarian!

Many of you don't know where the chlorine dioxide movement started over 30 years ago. It started with my great friend, Jim Humble.

My dear friend Jim. I can't believe the time has come to say goodbye forever. The 2 years you lived with me as part of my family will forever be etched in my heart and mind. As I promised you in February 2011, when I went to the Dominican Republic to thank you for the answers to my prayers to heal autism, I told you that I would do the same as you have done. Here I am after 13 years this 2023 with more than 100,000 people knowing that there is a solution to heal autism and that you brought it to us, the masses. You are a true humanitarian. I am grateful to have been able to meet your children Paris and James. I am very sorry for their loss as well. And your beautiful and loving wife of 10 years, Cari. She took good care of you. Always making sure you were handsome and neat. She will miss you too. My heart is broken. This news seems so definitive. I hope you carry in your heart how much I love you and always will. You are one of the greatest blessings in my life. Forever and always. Your friend and family member of the heart.

Kerri Rivera

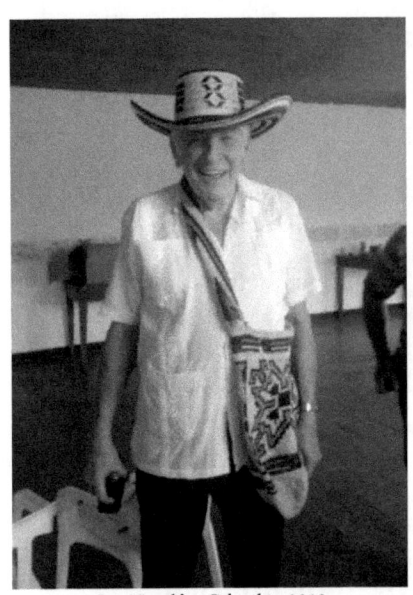
Jim Humble - Colombia 2012

On September 5, 2023, I received the terrible, terrible news that my great friend Jim Humble passed away on September 1, 2023. I have put off making the video for social media for a while because I am having a very hard time with the news. It's not so easy to talk about someone who did so much for so many and was someone very close to me. Some of you will know that he was close to me, but many of you will not. Jim Humble lived with me and my family from 2012-2014.

He lived a long life. He was going to be 91 this December 2023. He had a great life. He was a great person. He was always a very open person. He was stubborn, he had his likes and dislikes. He was willing to help anyone. That was definitely, I would say, the unique thing about this legend. And he was a living legend for the last 30 years, having founded chlorine dioxide (CD) for health and healing, which he called MMS. And he was very protective of calling it MMS. So, when I wrote my first book on CD 11 years ago (2013) and I said, I think we should call it chlorine dioxide because MMS is just a nickname for it, and he was like, no, I spent all these years calling it MMS. And of course, the world knows about MMS anyway, so he was very proud of his work, and he should be, because he took chlorine dioxide in its nickname "MMS" to the world. There is probably not a living being who has not heard of MMS at some level. He was a great friend and my heart longs for him. He was very much like a father to me.

He was someone who I am very grateful to have met, known and to have been able to live with and wake up to and see at breakfast, lunch and dinner with him and everything else between from 2012 and 2014. I would also like to offer my condolences to his wife Cari, whom he met at a conference we did in Puerto Vallarta, Mexico, in 2013. She took wonderful care of him and was a great wife and partner to Jim. She is a beautiful woman. So, he was able to see a beautiful and kind person throughout that last decade of his life. He had two children, Paris, and James, with his first wife when he was very young, also following in their father's footsteps, very intelligent and kind. Paris and James took a cruise that passed through Puerto Vallarta where we liked at the time. We got to spend a whole day with them, which was absolutely wonderful to be able to get to know them. He only had two children in his life, although he had several wives. He had had five wives in total. But of course, Jim was a person who let people be. He was not a person who would fight. He was a very good person, a very, very good person. The kind of person you rarely meet. I really haven't met someone like Jim before nor after since him in my entire life. He was so unique. And I'm very grateful that he had Carl Lloyd, his last wife. She's actually written books with him, and those last ten years he really did quite a bit. And he was always so proud of the legacy he had left in the world. He knew it and was able to enjoy that.

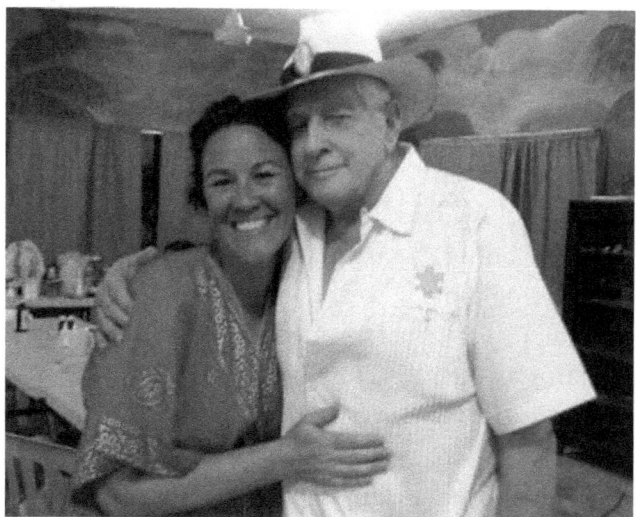

Kerri Rivera and Jim Humble in Dominican Republic, February 2011.

There are many people with legacies who don't know about it before they die and aren't really able to enjoy it. And that was one of the things with Jim that he was able to enjoy what he created. His legacy was left to people like Andreas Kalcker, myself, Mark Grenon and the Grenon family. And we know that many of us have paid a high price for the way the USA government persecutes people who promote things that are inexpensive and useful and healing that solve many of the world's problems. I first came across chlorine dioxide "MMS" in 2009, purchasing it from a doctor in Mexico. I didn't use it until 2010. I didn't know how to use it. So, I emailed Jim Humble, and received no response. Finally, after a few days, I received an email from Mark Grenon. He said, "I'll tell Jim to send you an email." Jim provided me with some very limited dosing for kids. He said if the child is 25lb then give 1 drop 8 x a day, if the child is 50lbs then give 2 drops 8 times a day. And if the child is 100lbs to give 3 drops 8 times a day. There was nothing on the internet about how to CD/MMS for children, much less children with autism. But when I looked on the internet, there was a ton of information about how to use it to kill viruses, bacteria, candida, parasites and how it helps to neutralize heavy metals. It reduces overall inflammation from the body. All this is known to be autism. I knew I was on the right track. That was in August 2010. So between August 2010 when I first used CD/MMS for autism and early October 2011, more than 40 lost their autism diagnosis, that is, they recovered from autism.

So, in January of 2011, I said, I have to go to the Dominican Republic and meet this very honorable man and give him a hug and thank him for bringing chlorine dioxide to the light of day. Because finally there was a solution for autism which seemed to have no solution. I met with Jim in the Dominican Republic in February 2011. I made a PowerPoint presentation about the CD autism protocol that I created for a workshop they were doing there. I met a lot of nice people there and remain friends with some of them to this day. And of course, I stayed in touch with Jim Humble. And then, in November 2011, when I returned to the Dominican Republic for the last time, to thank him again, as more and more children were recovered from autism.

Especially because of Venezuela and the foundation in Venezuela where they served thousands of children with my CD protocol. Many more children had lost their autism diagnosis. And at that time, the Dominican Republic was kind of falling out of favor with Jim, and he was ready to move on for many reasons. Nothing to do with the people that he was with, but it had more to do with the place itself. So, I asked him "Why don't you come live with me and my family in Puerto Vallarta, Mexico"? We have an extra bedroom. He accepted!!! And so, he lived with us for two years. And like I said, these years were so special, because he was just a special human being.

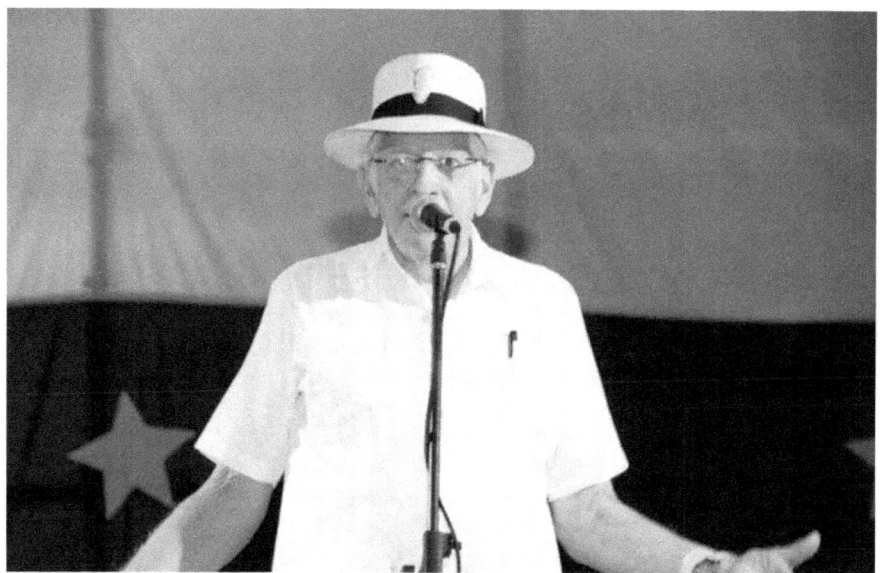

Jim Humble in Venezuela, October 2012

During those 2 years, we traveled together to Venezuela and Colombia. We held conferences and workshops in Colombia, Mexico as well as in the Czech Republic. We met so many like-minded people. In the last workshop in Puerto Vallarta Mexico is where Jim met his last wife, Cari, with whom he spent his last eleven of his life till his death. She was a wonderful person. The last time I saw them both was in Berlin, March of 2017. There was a conference celebrating Jim's 25-year Jubilee with CD/MMS.

The conference was organized by Leo Koehof, rest in peace. Also, a man who did a lot for Jim Humble and the entire chlorine dioxide movement. Leo did the Red Cross malaria study in Africa for CD/MMS. At the conference Jim gave a speech. It was probably the last one he gave. It was great to see him on stage talking about chlorine dioxide and his journey. Jim was a guy who loved his Pepsi Cola. He didn't like Coca Cola. He loved his coffee with cream and sugar. Jim could have coffee with cream and sugar at any time of the day or night and never passed up a chocolate cake. He liked chocolate. He didn't drink alcohol. He didn't like it. Those were just the things he most liked. He liked simple things. He was from Alabama, which is a state in the south of the USA. He was very American in certain aspects such as his diet. And he had some interesting sayings that always stay with me, and they make me smile. One of them was, "if it ain't broke, don't fix it." And it seems so simple, but it's so profound.

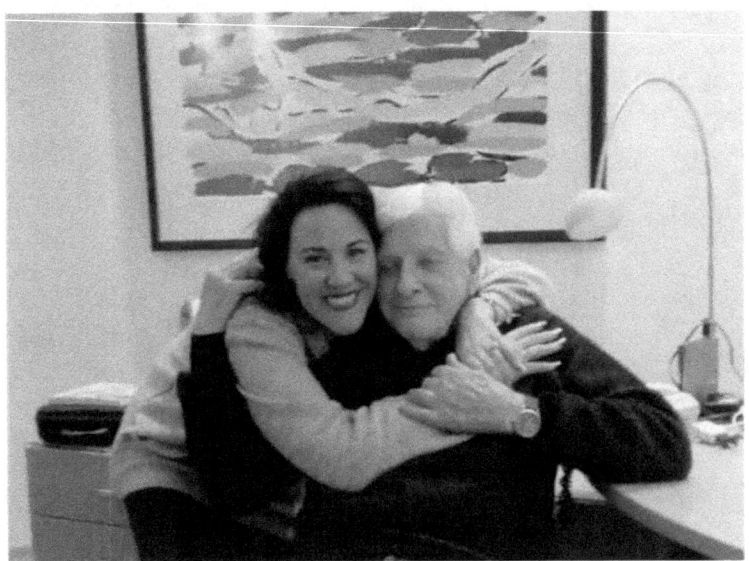

Kerri Rivera and Jim Humble in Berlin, 2017.

That has always stuck with me. It makes absolute sense to me that if the things are working why would anyone try to change them or fix them? He used to say, "WOWWWWWW" if he liked something or if it were a surprise. It was the way he said it that always made me laugh.

And he called most women "SWEETIE" because he had a terrible memory for names. That was Jim, he was terrible with names. And I think the only reason he remembered my name was because his last wife was named Cari, and his first wife was Terry. So, he remembered my name. Jim discovered the health benefits of CD/MMS while on a gold mining expedition in South America. He was a miner and people were getting malaria in the mining camps including his. He had bought the CD/MMS drops to make the water drinkable from a camping store in the USA before going on the trip. He thought, well, if you take the CD/MMS and you can kill pa\thogens in water to make it potable. Why couldn't the people collapsing from malaria drink it to kill the malaria in their bodies. And that's exactly what happened. He became very popular for his discovery. So popular that he was then invited to Africa to see if it would work for HIV/AIDS. This is part of where Leo Keoff came in. He did the study with the Red Cross against malaria, where 54 out of 54 people who tested positive for malaria in Africa were negative for malaria the next day. Then from Africa he moved to Mexico with a family who began to sell CD/MMS. From there he went to live in the Dominican Republic with Mark Grenon and his family doing workshops and training people on how to use the CD/MMS for health and healing. This is when Jim's message of health and healing began to spread far and wide.

Jim was a true was a living legend. This was carried forward by Mark Grenon and his family because they were able to do these workshops and train others to train. Jim and Mark traveled around the world training people in workshops. And then, in 2012, he moved permanently to Mexico, where he died on September 1, 2023, he was with his wife, Cari Lloyd. That's how Jim moved through the world. I would have loved to have been able to tell him before he passed away that his legend lives on in us. My dear friend Jim, I love you very much and you will always be in my heart. I will never forget you. And I am so grateful for the time we spent together and the projects we did together, the laughter we shared and, of course, the joy of being able to spread the word that there are solutions to the world's problems and that people don't have to suffer.

You were an incredible person, an incredible friend, a mentor, and you are always with me in my heart and work. Thank you for everything you did, my dear friend. Rest in peace. I love you very much.

Chapter 13
Voices of Hope
Parents' Stories about Their Children's Changes

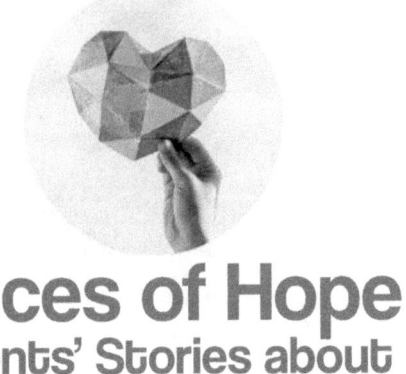

Voices of Hope
Parents' Stories about
Their Children's Changes

"Hi Kerri and team!

I am extremely excited to have the opportunity to address you. I've been wanting to do it for a long time, and I will take advantage of the invitation on Telegram to give my testimony for the book. My name is Gemma Campa, I am 48 years old, and I live in Tampico, Tamaulipas, Mexico. I am a single mother of a 9-year-old boy named Aidan Varg Campa.

Let me be brief, although my journey here has been full of experiences and anecdotes. Before Varg was born, I had a fetal doppler study, and the doctor told me that the baby was doing perfectly well. He even showed me the star-shaped cerebral cortex, explaining that this indicated that the baby was completely healthy, well formed and responding to stimuli. When he was born, everything seemed to be in order. I breastfed him for a couple of days, but then on the third day we took him to get vaccinated as directed by the doctor, and after that he didn't want me to breastfeed him anymore. Little by little, I began to notice that he was a very calm child, even though he cried and laughed, but I didn't pay much attention to it, thinking it was part of his temperament.

As time passed and we completed the required vaccinations, Varg began to lose abilities. He stopped eating many things he used to enjoy, developed allergies, and suffered frequent infections. He stopped babbling and retired to a corner of the room, where he spent hours without wanting to leave. These are just some examples of what was happening. The pediatrician told me that it was normal and that I should give him time to start talking. However, the daycare director noticed several problems in his development and advised me to seek professional help. At first, I rejected it, thinking it was just a passing phase, but when the director insisted that I needed help, I began to worry. The psychologist we consulted did not provide a clear answer about Varg's condition but indicated a delay in his psychosocial development. I was frustrated as I couldn't get a definitive answer about what was happening to my son.

The situation became even more complicated with the arrival of the pandemic. I lost my job, we were housebound, and my son slept only an hour a day and up to six hours at night. Then, I found a video by a woman from Colombia, in which she said that her son had overcome autism. At first, I didn't believe it, but I decided to take action and eliminate wheat, milk, Play-Doh compounds and Heinz brand aluminum canned baby food from Varg's diet. This happened in 2020. Additionally, I started giving him essential oils, which I believe helped keep my son stable and prevent him from getting worse.

By 2022, I began to awaken to a new understanding and became aware of the manipulation of our cognitive processes by the elites. I then discovered Dr. Bayter and eliminated fruits and vegetable oils from our daily diet, which caused my son to start sleeping properly. Then, in a moment of reflection and gratitude, I said the name "Andres" to express my gratitude for my son's health. Later, I discovered that I had pronounced "Andreas," not "Andres," and that this was related to the answer I needed for my son's health. In less than 24 hours, I had Andreas' protocol, the chlorine dioxide (CDS) and everything I needed to start the treatment. As I did more research and found peace of mind, I decided to switch from Andreas' protocol to Kerri's protocol. Over the past three months, I have noticed significant improvements, especially with the transition from CDS to CD, which has helped my son stop having daily meltdowns due to the sound of the train since we live so close to the tracks.

One of the biggest challenges has been changing my son's eating habits and confronting the family about this. We faced the wrath of some doctors and ridicule from people close to us. I now understand that humanity is conditioned and that we often have a preconceived negative perspective. This makes us hesitate when we are told about a cure that does not come from a "professional" or someone in a white coat. When they explain to us and demonstrate that something works, we fall into cognitive dissonance. It is evident that staying in the bubble of accepting our children's condition, dictated by a corrupt industry, often seems more comfortable than unlearning and embarking on a new path of knowledge, routine and the uncertainty of how our children will react. At least that's what happened to me.

When my son Varg started the protocol in July 2022, his ATEC score was 99. He did not maintain eye contact, he ignored everyone, he did not speak, he only repeated numbers and letters of the alphabet, he isolated himself in a corner of the house, he had allergies, a bloated abdomen, sensitivity to loud noises, he hit his face and screamed for no apparent reason. Today, October 7, 2023, his ATEC score has decreased to 30. He now looks me in the eyes when I talk to him, meets my gaze, and tries to formulate sentences to communicate. He laughs and seeks the company of other children, he greets people when he sees them, he has stopped hitting himself and can control himself better when faced with loud noises. He also follows instructions at school and breaks routines on his own initiative. The most important decision I have made was to follow my instinct and not pay attention to the opinions of others, and this has been possible thanks to the CD protocol by Kerri Rivera. We are a testament to the hard work of Kerri Rivera, Andreas Kalcker and Jim Humble. We thank you for giving us your unconditional love through this knowledge. But most of all, Kerri, you are in the constant care of thousands of families, we appreciate you very much. You are a beautiful being and an example as a mother for me and for many people. THANK YOU!

I share some photos so you can get to know my Aidan Varg before the protocol and during it. Thank you, Kerri, and team, I send you a huge hug and lots of love."

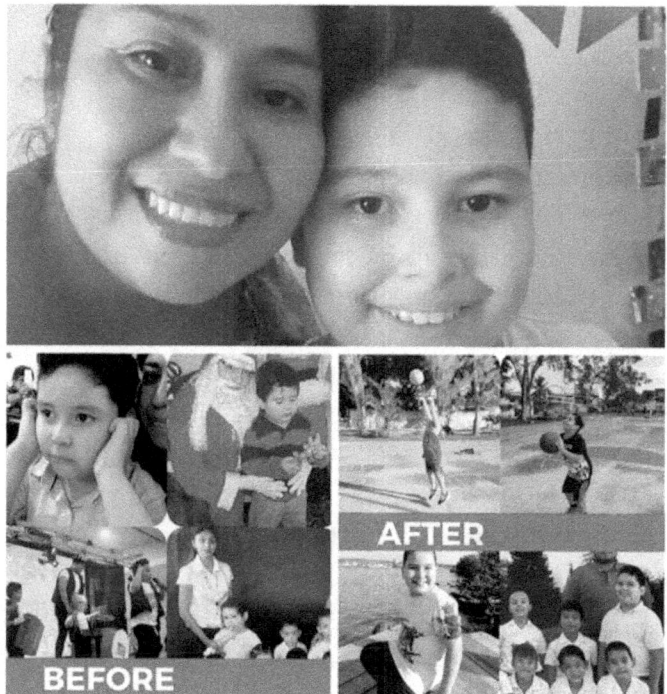

"Thank you so much, Kerri really! I am aware of everything that happens around you and of all those who tell the truth and threaten the system, but we will not comply, and we will find a way to spread your voice. When it comes to autism, you are the teacher of teachers! (The mother of ice cream as we say in Venezuela) I know because I have searched all over the world and we have a saying at home that says, "all roads lead to Kerri.""

User: Sebnem

Hello, Kerri. Thank you, my son has improved a lot with your protocol, today the speech therapist reduced my son's class schedule, oh my god she is improving only her side glances and her speech as her classmates remained Teşekkürler Keri Rivera Teşekkürler Andreas Teşekkürler Jim Humble

User: The_Rolling_Stone

"Hello good morning. I wanted to tell you about my 3-year-old son Otto. He is outside the autism spectrum. He was evaluated yesterday by his 2 neurologists and an ASD specialist. And do you know why that is? Thanks to the CD and Kerri Rivera. 1 year already in this group. With many struggles. Because my son didn't want to take the CD. He would spit it at me, he would kick me if I wanted to give it to him. I had to force him... Nowadays he does the CD doses without crying. He takes his 18 drops. Sometimes he doesn't want to, and it is understandable that he is tired of it. But he takes it anyway. There is no problem with the diet. Otto was a boy who only ate noodles, oats, and milk. He didn't want anyone to get close to him. He would lie on the floor for more than 1 hour. He was afraid of babies. He cried and screamed. He hit me and hit himself and much more. Today he is a boy who has friends. That goes to the garden. He plays with his cousins. He recognizes his dad when he comes to visit. He loves music, the squares and going to theaters to see Zenón's farm or see someone sing. That used to bother him a lot. I can go to work calmly because he behaves very well and stays with my mother. He loves his books, loves to draw, and paint. He leads a normal life and that makes me happy. What we have to improve now is his language so he can form more than 2 sentences. With his speech therapy and more protocol, he will. He was totally mute. Now he tells me "Mom, come. give me water. I don't want to. Let's go there, etc..." We have to continue. So, cheer up and continue. Because all this is true and with each passing day we will recover more of our children. It also helped me a lot to talk to parents in this group who were always very good to me. And I am super grateful." God bless you!!!

User: Gaby Vergara

"Hello everyone. I would like to share my testimony; I have an 8-year-old girl. We have been using the protocol for 6 months and it has gone very well! Last year my daughter showed very alarming behaviors that she had never had before, until we found Kerri's protocol, and we knew that these behaviors could be PANDAS, we informed ourselves well, we studied the guide for parents over and over again and with great faith and wanting to help her, we started the protocol. My daughter's initial ATEC was 98 then 64 and now we are at 48 and going for more! Seriously, parents, don't despair, don't give up, it's difficult, yes, but as the months go by and there are improvements in behaviors and symptoms, every effort, every battle is totally worth it! Until now the strongest battle has been against the symptoms of PANDAS. We still have a way to go and we are sure that we will do even better! If possible!! Much encouragement, perseverance and patience. Many thanks to Kerri for this excellent treatment" Blessings to all!

User: Laurien NM

"I am a witness that really more than a specialist, she is a mother committed to helping families heal the bodies of children from autism. All my respect to you (Kerri Rivera) and to my dear Carolina. God bless you with so much love for returning my son to us, who was also lost in the bubble of autism.

Jesús David made his first communion, he is now in third grade. He is a child who is developing like a typical child. He laughs, cries, expresses himself, hugs, is sociable, asks a lot of questions, tells me that when he is an adult, he wants to get married and have children. One day he wants to be a YouTuber, another day a Police Officer, God will put his real vocation in his heart. I owe this to God and Kerri Rivera. Blessings."

User: Mayda

"Good morning, my girl with autism is 5 years and 6 months old. 17

days ago, we started on the low glutamate diet, chlorine dioxide (CD) and CD enemas, ultra blinder, H-7 formula and pekticlean. Since last week she began sleeping through the night without waking up until 7am. She is non-verbal, but she has begun to babble more, for the first time this week she performed well in her speech therapy. She began to communicate better by pointing out what she wants and has been calmer. Yesterday we went to a restaurant, and she stayed seated the entire time. We are so happy to see so many changes in such a short period of time. God willing it will continue like this. Many thanks to Kerri Rivera and her team"

User: Gverow

"Good morning. I wanted to deeply thank Kerri for her generosity in sharing her protocols. My 9-year-old boy with non-verbal autism has started talking!!!!! Very little by little he uses words in a communicative way. God bless her greatly."

CHEER UP! IT'S POSSIBLE!

"It is important when we see a path in front of us that seems long and impossible. That we remember that more than 100,000 people since 2010 have done my protocol. If it were possible to do so many times before, you too can do it. Remember, you are the only advocate for your child that exists. RECOVERY IS POSSIBLE! Never give up. Never let negative thoughts enter your mind. Remember that thousands of children have recovered with this protocol. Assume that your child is going to be one of them. Protocols for autism must include detoxing the body from pathogens. Not by doing lab testing and then filling the children full of vitamins. CD protocol works because the focus is on recovery by treating the underlying causes that are labeled "autism". I hope and pray for a full and fast recovery for every child. You have come to the right place since you have read this book till here.
Kerri

Chapter 14
Contact with Kerri

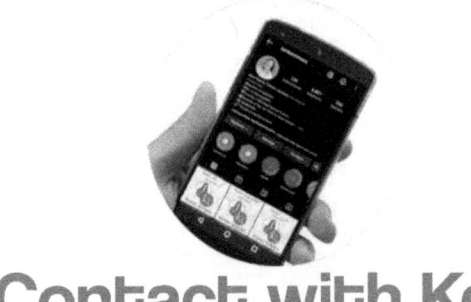

Contact with Kerri

How to schedule a consultation with Kerri?

1. Place your order at **www.kerririvera.com**
2. Then send an email to **kerri@kerririvera.com** with the following information:
   - » Number of order
   - » Child's name
   - » Age
   - » Weight
   - » Parents name
   - » Country
   - » Time zone
   - » Skype account
   - » Email

3. Consultations are carried out via video call.
4. If you do not receive a response regarding the day and time of your inquiry within the next 48 hours, please contact the support team at:cdautismosoporte@gmail.com
5. Due to censorship, I do not receive emails from **Yahoo! Hotmail, AOL, icloud, Rogers among many others, nor am I able to send them.** They have blocked and censored me. Instead, we recommend opening an email account at **Gmail or better yet it is ProtonMail.** To make sure that you are able to stay in contact with Kerri.

6. Consultations are available in: Spanish, English, Italian and Portuguese.
7. When you have questions about products. Feel free to send me an email to help you find what we are using. Sometimes we have to speak in code because of censorship. It's a drag. This is proof that we are over the target.

Kerri's email:
  » kerri@kerririvera.com

Telegram Support Groups in Spanish:
  » t.me/cdautismo
  » t.me/krdietas
  » t/mekerririvera2022

Telegram Support Groups in English:
  » t.me/iamkerririvera

Kerri's social networks inInstagram and Tiktok:
  » @iamkerririvera

In case the social media censor us again at some point. Send me an email at **kerri@kerririvera.com** and I will help you to find the support groups. In February of 2019, I had over 60,000 people in my Facebook groups in 13 different languages. Overnight, Facebook deleted all the groups, and they froze my personal account as well. You can still see my account, yet I have no way to access it nor answer private messages should someone send me one. It is possible that one day the same thing will happen on Telegram or Instagram. But my email is my own and I have my own computer server so that is the best place to find me if we lose touch.

About the Author

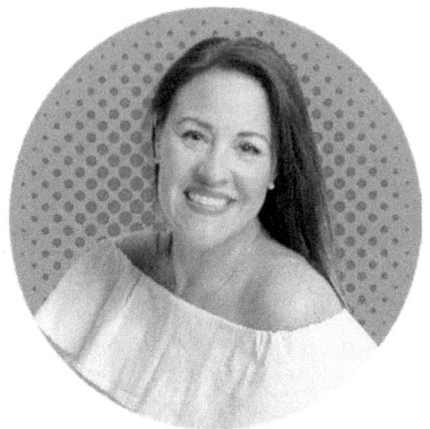

Kerri Rivera is a leading autism expert with a solid track record with more than 20 years of experience. She is a homeopath and certified clinician in the DAN approach! (Defeat Autism Now), specializing in biomedical treatments and hyperbaric oxygen therapy (HBOT). She is a trained hyperbaric technician. In addition to this, she is the author of several books as well as an international speaker and a reference in the field of autism.

As the founder and director of the first biomedical autism treatment clinic in Latin America, her innovative approach challenges conventional perspectives by addressing the medical causes of autism. Her strong training and clinical certifications support her approach, and she has transformed lives and brought hope to numerous families seeking real solutions.

With a proven track record of success working with tens of thousands of children with autism, Kerri Rivera has demonstrated her commitment and exceptional skills in delivering tangible results in the field of autism.

REFERENCES

- Agarwal SP, Khanna R, Karmarkar R, Anwer MK, Khar RK (2007). Shilajit: a review. Phytother Res 2007; 21: 401–405.
- Burlakovs J, Klavins M, Osinska L, Purmalis O (2013). The Impact of Humic Substances as Remediation Agents to the Speciation Forms of Metals in Soil. APCBEE Procedia Volume 5, 2013, Pages 192-196.
- Campbell, Keith (2016). "Over 40 minerals and metals contained in seawater, their extraction likely to increase in the future," Creamer's Media Mining Weekly. https://www.miningweekly.com/article/over-40-minerals-and-metals-contained-in-seawater-their- extraction-likely-to-increase-in-the-future-2016-04-01
- Chopra RN, Chopra, I.C., Handa, K.L., Kapur, L.D. Chopra's Indigenous drugs of india, 2nd ed. B Calcutta India; K Dhur of academic Publishers. 1958.
- Dekker J, Medlen CE, inventor (2003). Oxihumic acid and its use in the treatment of the various conditions.
- Ghosal S, Lal J, Singh SK (1991). The core structure of Shilajit humus. Soil Biology Biochem 23:673–680.
- Ghosal S (1993). Shilajit: Its origin and vital significance. In Traditional Medicine, Mukherjee B (ed.). Oxford – IBH: New Delhi, 308–319.
- Hess, M; Jones, RG; Kahovec, J; Kitayama, T; Kratochvil, P; Kubisa, P; Mormann, W; Stepto, RFT; Tabak, D; Vohlidal, J; Wilks, ES (2006). Pure Appl. Chem. Vol. 78, No. 11, pp. 2067– 2074.
- Hils J, May A, Sperber M, Klocking R, Helbig B, Sprossig M (1986). Inhibition of several strains of influenza virus type A and B by phenolic polymers. Biomed Biochim Acta 45:1173–1179.
- Kochany, J & Smith, W (2001). Application of humic substances in environmental remediation. Proceedings of WM'01 Conference, February 25–March 1, WM Symposia Inc., Tucson, AZ, USA.
- Laub RJ. (1999). Process for preparing synthetic soil-extract materials and medicaments based thereon. USA Patent 5,945,446.

- Mauizio Z., inventor (2002). Treatment of HIV infection with Humic acid. Paris.
- Meena H., Pandey H. K., Arya M. C., Ahmed Z. (2010). Shilajit: a panacea for high-altitude problems. International Journal of Ayurveda Research. 1(1):37–40. doi: 10.4103/0974- 7788.59942.
- Pandey, A.; Soccol, C. R.; Nigam, P.; Soccol, V. T.; Vandenberghe, L. P. S.; Mohan, R. (2000). Biotechnological potential of agro-industrial residues. II: cassava bagasse. Bioresource Technol., 74 (1): 81-87.
- Pant, Kishor & Singh, B & Thakur, Nagendra. (2012). Shilajit: A humic matter panacea for cancer. International Journal of Toxicological and Pharmacological Research. 4. 17-25.
- Peña-Méndez, EM, Havel, J, Patočka J. (2005). Humic substances—compounds of still unknown structure: applications in agriculture, industry, environment, and biomedicine. Appl Biomed. 3:13-24.
- Pettit RE (2004). Organic matter, humus, humate, humic acid, fulvic acid and humin: their importance in soil fertility and plant health [Online]. https://humates.com/pdf/ORGANICMATTER-Pettit.pdf
- Riede UN, Zeck-Kapp G, Freudenberg N, Keller HU, Seubert B. (1991). Humate-induced activation of human granulocytes. Virchows Arch B Cell Pathol Incl Mol Pathol 60:27–34.
- Schepetkin I, Khlebnikov A, Kwon BS. (2002). Medical Drugs from Humus Matter: Focus on Mumie. Drug Dev Res.; 57:140–159.
- Schepetkin IA, Khlebnikov AI, Ah SY, Woo SB, Jeong CS, Klubachuk ON, Kwon BS (2003). Characterization and Biological Activities of Humic Substances from Mumie. J Agric Food Chem; 51:5245-54.
- Schiller F., Klocking R, Wutzler P, Farber I. (1979). Results of an oriented clinical trial of ammonium humate for the local treatment of herpesvirus hominis (HVH) infections. Dermatol Monatsschr 165:505–509.
- Schnitzer M., Khan SU. (1972). Humic substances in the environment. New York: Marcel Dekker.
- Shenyuan Yuan, et al. (1993). Application of Fulvic acid and its derivatives in the fields of agriculture and medicine. 1st ed.

- Thiel KD, Klocking R, Schweizer H, Sprossig M. (1977). In vitro studies of the antiviral activity of ammonium humate against herpes simplex virus type 1 and type 2. Zentralbl Bakteriol A 239:304–321.
- Thiel KD, Helbig B, Klocking R, Wutzler P, Sprossig M, Schweizer, H. (1981). Comparison of the in vitro activities of ammonium humate and of enzymically oxidized chlorogenic and caffeic acids against type 1 and type 2 human herpes virus. Pharmazie 36: 50–53.
- van Rensburg CE, van Straten A, Dekker J. (2000). An in vitro investigation of the antimicrobial activity of oxifulvic acid. J Antimicrob Chemother 46:853.
- van Rensburg CE, Malfeld SCK, Dekker J. (2001). Topical application of oxifulvic acid suppresses the cutaneous immune response in mice. Drug Dev Res 53:29–32.
- Wang C, Wang Z, Peng A, Hou J, Xin W. (1996). Interaction between fulvic acids of different origins and active oxygen radicals. Sci China C Life Sci 39:267–275.
- Wilson E, Rajamanickam GV, Dubey GP, Klose P, Musial F, Saha, F, Rampp Thomas, Michalsen A, Dobos G (2011). Review on shilajit used in traditional Indian medicine. Journal of ethnopharmacology. 136. 1-9. 10.1016/j.jep.2011.04.033.
- Winkler, John; Ghosh, Sanjoy (2018). "Therapeutic Potential of Fulvic Acid in Chronic Inflammatory Diseases and Diabetes," Journal of Diabetes Research, vol. 2018, Article ID 5391014, 7 pages. https://doi.org/10.1155/2018/5391014.
- Yamauchi, Masashige; Katayama, Sadamu; Todoroki, Toshiharu; Watanable, Toshio (1984). "Total synthesis of fulvic acid". Journal of the Chemical Society, Chemical Communications (23): 1565–6. doi:10.1039/C39840001565.

PARENT GUIDE

Empowering parents on the road to recovery from autism. Kerri Rivera's step-by-step protocol by Kerri Rivera for you.

Kerri RIvera is a homeopath, DAN! clinician (Biomedical Treatments/Defeat Autism Now), hyperbaric technician, author of several books, international speaker and autism expert with over 20 years of experience.

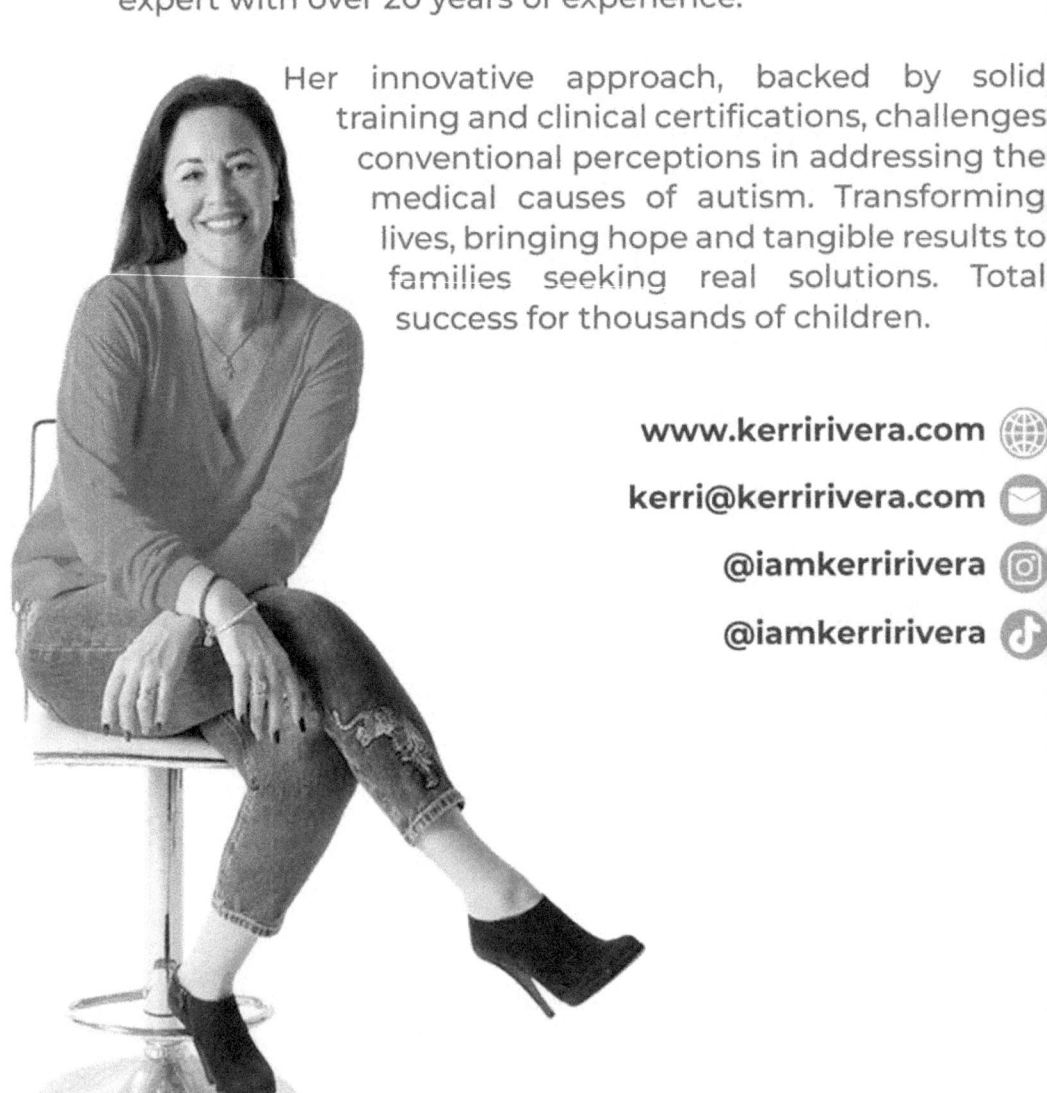

Her innovative approach, backed by solid training and clinical certifications, challenges conventional perceptions in addressing the medical causes of autism. Transforming lives, bringing hope and tangible results to families seeking real solutions. Total success for thousands of children.

www.kerririvera.com

kerri@kerririvera.com

@iamkerririvera

@iamkerririvera